TAKING CONTROL OF YOUR HEADACHES

TAKING CONTROL
OF YOUR
HEADACHES

How to Get the Treatment You Need

Paul N. Duckro, Ph.D.
William D. Richardson, M.D.
Janet E. Marshall, R.N.
with Steven Cassabaum and Greg Marshall

✦

Foreword by Seymour Diamond, M.D.

THE GUILFORD PRESS
New York   London

© 1995 The Guilford Press
A Division of Guilford Publications, Inc.
72 Spring Street, New York, NY, 10012

Printed in the United States of America

This book is printed on acid-free paper.

Last digit is print number: 9 8 7 6 5 4 3 2 1

Library of Congress Cataloging-in-Publication Data

Duckro, Paul N.
    Taking control of your headaches: how to get the treatment you need
/ by Paul N. Duckro, William D. Richardson, Janet E. Marshall; with
Steven Cassabaum and Greg Marshall
        p.   cm.
    Includes bibliographical references and index.
    ISBN 0-89862-787-7
    1. Headache—Popular works.   I. Richardson, William D., M.D.
II. Marshall, Janet E.   III. Title.
    RB128.D83 1995
    616.8'491—dc20   95-9413
                                                                   CIP

✦

Foreword

In this current era of "infomercials" and self-help courses, the public has been inundated with books on understanding and managing pain disorders, particularly headaches. Many of these books have been adequate, but many more have been unsatisfactory in some way. It was therefore a relief and a privilege to have the opportunity to read this book, *Taking Control of Your Headaches.*

For decades, the headache sufferer has felt confined to a closet; afraid that his or her headache problem will be exposed. Unfortunately, families and friends often considered headache to be a psychosomatic problem, or some other unacceptable disorder, and the victim to be a malingerer. However, public opinion over the past 20 years has changed, and pain problems, including headache, have been recognized as tangible disorders. This bias has changed in large part because of the pioneering efforts of the National Headache Foundation, which facilitated the public's realization and acceptance that headache is a valid disorder and requires adequate care.

During my 40 years of clinical experience in the management of headache I have evaluated many patients who have undergone a variety of interventions. Occasionally, these therapies are based on reason. However, in many instances, patients are needlessly exposed to unproven methodologies and countless machinations in the quest for relief. The litany of treatments seems endless. Patients have reported allergies desensitized, eyes refracted, eye muscles changed via exercise or surgery, vertebrae manipulated, uteri removed, hormones regulated, nerves injected or severed, holes drilled, trigger points punctured, sinuses drained, and septums undeviated. It is not unusual for patients to describe prolonged psychotherapy, hypnosis, and marriage counseling. The list of medical therapies is often compounded by dental intervention, including teeth extracted or straightened, fillings replaced, and the temporomandibular joints replaced or manipulated. Headache sufferers have extolled the virtues of exotic diets, herbs, yoga, and homeopathy. The irony of these treatments is that, in most instances, patients have been subject to one or more without attempts at a comprehensive approach, such as that delineated in this book.

Appropriate headache management must start with a thorough headache history that will usually require several hours. Diagnosis will be established through information gleaned from the history and complete physical and neurological examinations, as well as whatever testing is deemed necessary to rule out an organic disorder as the cause. Once this process is completed, diagnosis will become evident in most cases, enabling appropriate therapy to be selected.

For a migraine sufferer experiencing about one headache per month, one could deduce that abortive migraine medications would be more appropriate than years of counseling. Too often, however, patients encounter specialists or therapists who project their own agenda, and thereby victimize the patient with a myriad of therapies that reap no benefit. Such blatant excesses of treatment modalities are common. Headache sufferers should realize that the best approach to relief may be the simplest. This book gives insight into simple yet effective therapies and helps prevent pitfalls commonly associated with chronic headache treatment. It also affords a thorough understanding of headache symptoms and how readers can easily classify headache problems. The chapters on triggers, risk factors, and medications particularly enlighten patients as they attempt to relieve their pain. Many readers will readily appreciate the description of nondrug therapies that are presented throughout this book. (I must reiterate, however, that a multimodal approach is requisite, and drug therapy may be a necessary part of it.)

Because of my long tenure as a headache specialist, I have especially enjoyed this text and its advocacy of a multimodal, practical approach to headache problems. My delight in preparing this foreword is augmented by my long experience with one of the authors, Paul N. Duckro, Ph.D. Together, Paul and I have consulted and shared ideas, theories, and therapies. Dr. Duckro has actively served as both a consultant and editor of the journal *Headache Quarterly: Current Treatment and Research.* His hands-on approach to the headache patient is evident in this book. I am proud and honored to have been afforded the opportunity to add to this scholarly yet useful book. Readers, whether headache suffers or not, will gain from the insight expressed by these authors.

Seymour Diamond, M.D.
Diamond Headache Clinic
The Chicago Medical School
University of Medicine
and Dentistry of New Jersey

✦

Acknowledgments

N o project of this size can be accomplished without many hands. There are more people to whom we are indebted than we can possibly mention here. Thanks to every one of them.

We would like to mention especially Barbara Watkins, whose initial support was critical in moving our manual toward publication; Christine Benton, whose tireless assistance shaped the language and presentation of the material; Mary Franklin, whose generous review of an earlier draft was invaluable; Dr. Seymour Diamond, whose clinical mentoring has taught us so much; our colleagues at St. Louis University whose insights and efforts have helped our many patients; our families, without whose support nothing else would happen; and our patients themselves, whose courage, honesty, and observations have inspired and educated us all.

We hope this book, in what it will give to others, is some recompense for all that we have been given.

✦

Contents

Introduction

Ⅰf you have chronic headaches, you know how one feels—how it squeezes, burns, pounds, drills. You know what it brings with it, from nausea to sleeplessness to irritability. And you know how it leaves you feeling—like a victim, with less freedom in work and family life, less joy in living than you deserve. Too often the headache is in control. Instead of doing as you would truly like to, you wind up doing as the headache says you must.

More than 40 million people in the United States have severe headaches—headaches that disrupt their lives, making it difficult or impossible to carry out their normal routine at work or home—at least sometime in their lives. In one sense, most of these are also chronic headaches: very few are the result of a life-threatening medical disease. When they occur infrequently, perhaps once or twice per year, most people adjust to them. Unpleasant as they may be, life goes on normally most of the time. Sometimes, however, chronic severe headaches become more frequent, last for a long time, and become part of a person's routine every month, every week, or even every day. If you fit this description, you are among as many as 16 million Americans with the same problem. This book is written for you.

With proper diagnosis and the right medication, chronic headaches can sometimes be controlled. But what about those that cannot—those that do not respond to medication or respond at first but then seem to overpower the medicine that once worked so well? What about those headaches that actually begin to increase in frequency or severity even as medication use also increases and emergency room visits spiral? And what about instances when medication use, while helping to control the headaches, threatens to cause other health problems or to interfere with your ability to function on the job or at home? You may begin to wonder, or hear others wondering, if you really are a "junkie" seeking medication or you just have a low tolerance for pain. Your self-esteem may begin to fall, self-doubts to build.

These judgments are generally not valid, but clearly something more than just more or different medication is needed in such cases. We believe that a *multimodal approach* serves the chronic headache patient best. Multimodal treatment is just one name to describe the type of integrated treatment offered by headache specialists. It begins with thorough diagnosis—not just an array of tests but time to really listen to the story of the headache patient, what you have noticed about your own unique headache history. It continues with the use of a variety of treatments selected to fit your particular needs. Certainly this involves medication, but medication is not asked to carry the whole weight of management. Other treatments often include physical therapy and behavioral therapy and sometimes involve other dental and medical procedures as suggested by the diagnostic process. Behavioral therapy is itself a complex enterprise and is often an unexpected part of the treatment process to people with headaches. Multimodal treatment ends with regular follow-up in which you stay on the alert for the need to change medicine, keep up self-care, and catch relapses early. Perhaps best of all, it puts you back in control.

In multimodal therapy, you become a crucial member of the treatment team. The physicians, psychologists, and other professionals on your team help you learn what may be triggering your headaches and what you do to make them better or worse. They also provide tools you can use to reduce the impact of those factors identified as headache risks ("triggers" of headache) for you. Of course, this team cannot cure headache; that is not possible with our current knowledge. These professionals can help you manage headaches effectively. This does not mean just asking you to live with pain but really results in fewer headaches lasting for shorter periods of time. They cannot do the work for you, but they can show you the way and walk it with you. It may seem like much work, but it is effective, and it is empowering. You become part of the solution, not just a victim or sufferer.

Multimodal treatment is also the logical alternative when you find yourself unable to take medication because of its side effects, another illness, or pregnancy. Beyond these factors we suggest that any treatments that allow you to reduce your use of medication are simply reasonable choices. No medication is completely safe, and any medication taken in high doses or for a long time becomes more problematic. We all must continue to become better at taking care of ourselves, preventing disease, and using many sources of healing.

The principal aim of this book, therefore, is to put control of your headaches more firmly into your hands. You may use it for your own information and/or as a reference and an aid in working with your physician. Ideally, it can be a type of treatment manual, used as part of a comprehensive approach to treatment of your headaches with a competent headache treatment team. In the following chapters you will find up-to-date information on what professional help is available, how to find it, and how to use it to control your headaches and improve the quality of your life. Chapter 1 will help you get appropriate treatment by telling you what to expect from headache professionals and how to find them. Chapter 2 explains exactly how multimodal treatment works. In Chapter 3 you will learn about the major groups of headaches and how your treatment team tries to understand your symptoms in terms of these categories. Chapters 4 and 5 explain the many factors that can trigger headaches. The most widely used modes of therapy—medication, physical therapy, relaxation, and cognitive-behavioral therapy—are described in Chapters 6–9. Chapter 10 discusses special categories of headache not addressed separately earlier in the book. Throughout the book illustrative case studies elaborate on the multimodal process, and charts and checklists give you additional tools to manage your headaches.

While the entire book is aimed at answering *your* needs and concerns, we hope it will also be of use to family members and loved ones who wish to support your efforts and to headache professionals. Our patients use this book as a manual as they go through treatment at our facility, and other doctors and therapists may also find the book useful for their patients as a review of treatment strategies and, in combination with other books listed at the end of this book, as a general reference.

Our experience at the chronic headache clinic of the St. Louis University School of Medicine indicates that physicians as well as patients feel frustrated when medication-only treatment fails. Physicians want to help but are dissatisfied with prescribing more medication than may be healthy with little to show for it in the way of successful management of headaches. Patients begin to feel hopeless and helpless. They feel uncomfortable about their increasing use of medication but frightened of the consequences if they do not take it. Both are caught in a trap.

The answer for the chronic headache patient seldom lies with an esoteric treatment or an undiscovered rare disease. These things happen, but they are uncommon. The practitioner who is wedded to a single type of treatment for all headaches is likely to be the wrong person for you. As Abraham Maslow said, if the only tool you have is a hammer, everything starts to look like a nail. Typically, the approach that helps is a systematically applied combination of safe and reliable treatment techniques. Even when patients who come to us have tried all the methods we discuss here, most have not had them prescribed in an integrated program by a team that is really talking together.

What you will find summarized in this book is a sound and practical treatment regimen combining well-studied methods of therapy with real attention to the individual needs of the headache patient. The keys are flexibility, integration, coordination, and persistence. Flexibility allows the team to assess the particular patient in front of them and to suggest treatments from a whole range of possibilities. Integration is the use of medical, psychological, and physiological techniques to affect different aspects of the headache problem. Coordination means professionals who talk together and learn from each other and from their patients. Persistence is the willingness to stay with the problem, reviewing initial impressions and changing course if results are not forthcoming. This is the type of treatment found in a comprehensive headache clinic using multimodal treatment.

More Americans complain of headache than of any other kind of pain, yet many do not feel understood, listened to, or respected. Only about half are currently seeking professional help. Some suffer from migraine and never have it diagnosed; others have found simple treatments prescribed in their doctor's office ineffective, have stopped seeking help, and now try to handle their headaches on their own with over-the-counter (OTC) medications. Clinical experience suggests that as many as 90 percent of headache sufferers can find at least some relief through appropriate treatment. More than two-thirds of those who come to our clinic, even with very persistent and severe headaches that have not responded to other attempts at treatment, find multimodal treatment very helpful. They tell us they are glad they came. We hope you will be glad you bought this book and that it will help you regain hope that you can manage your headaches, find relief from your pain, and build renewed contentment and joy in everyday life.

✦

CHAPTER 1

Get the Help You Need

W hen should you seek professional help for headaches, and how do you go about finding it? Up to one-sixth of Americans suffer from severe headaches, yet a great number of them never seek help or never receive effective treatment. According to a study done by one of the authors in the late 1980s, almost 16 percent of adult heads of households surveyed in the St. Louis area had experienced some headaches severe enough to interfere with their daily routine. Many of these people had such headaches once a month or more often. Another study reported that more than half of migraine headache patients are undiagnosed, and still another showed that more than half of the migraine headache patients studied relied only on over-the-counter medication even for their very severe headaches. Obviously the United States is full of individuals suffering from chronic and severe headaches without optimal treatment.

This chapter tells you how to make a preliminary, general assessment of your own headaches and then how to get the necessary professional help to control the headaches.

WHEN TO GET HELP

Many people have headaches that are triggered by muscle tension and/or psychological stress. For most, the headache is relatively infrequent and mild; they just take a painkiller, the headache goes away, and they forget about it. Obviously if you fall into this group you do not need special care, though you should bring your headaches to the attention of your primary care physician in the course of ordinary checkups. Other people have very severe headaches, but they do not occur often. If you have these types of episodic headaches, see your doctor for a diagnosis; most episodic headaches can be treated with medication to cut the headaches short. A small group will experience an extremely severe headache—perhaps one they would describe as the worst headache they have ever had—relatively suddenly. Should this happen to you, you should see your doctor as soon as possible.

The group that can benefit most from the information in this book are those who have more frequent severe headaches. Severe headaches once or twice a month usually get your serious attention. The pain can be excruciating, and the toll on family life and job responsibilities is often significant. In this book we will call this syndrome *chronic headache*. Of course, strictly speaking, any headache that is not the result of a particular underlying disease can be called chronic, because there is no known cure. However, we are particularly concerned with severe headaches that occur more frequently over time, and that is what we mean when we discuss chronic headache in this book. Such severe headaches are, in effect, a chronic disease like any other. Diabetes is a good comparison. It cannot be cured, but it can be managed with proper medication and changes in behavior or lifestyle.

Chronic Daily Headache

Professionals vary in their definition of this term, and it is not yet an official diagnosis. When someone has headaches more than fifteen days a month, most clinicians begin to consider the problem a daily or near-daily headache. Some patients have headaches this frequently right from the beginning of their problem. More often the number of days on which headaches strike increases gradually. As we will see later in this book, there are different types of chronic daily headache as well.

Chronic daily headache can develop for many different reasons. For example, depression, commonly associated with chronic pain of any kind, including chronic headache, can play a negative role, making the pain more frequent and severe. Most of the time the depression seems to result from the pain, from a feeling of loss of control, and from the loss of many sources of ordinary pleasure and release. But even if depression is strictly the *result* of the pain rather than its cause, it can worsen chronic headache. Muscle tension can also contribute. When you have chronic pain such as headaches, you may tense in response to the headache or adopt poor postures in reaction to the pain; the resulting muscle irritation may then exacerbate the headaches. Complex medication regimens, sometimes self-directed, affect the body in unintended ways and may, paradoxically (explained further in Chapter 6), also perpetuate the headaches.

The way you think can also be a factor in turning chronic headache into chronic daily headache. Inevitably your thoughts may become trained on the seemingly ever-present headache, distracting you from factors that may be contributing to the problem. Whereas those with episodic headaches often recognize the role of stressful everyday events in their headaches, chronic headache patients tend to believe that everything would be fine if only they didn't have these headaches. Their ignorance of contributing causes over which they actually have some control ends up compounding the problem.

Finally, the stress of chronic pain can affect all your relationships. Family relations are ruined when one member is frequently out of commission, and job success is threatened by days off and reductions in efficacy. The stress resulting from this type of damage can do nothing but worsen the headache problem. Indeed all these factors may contribute to the development and maintenance of chronic daily headache.

While frequency of headaches is a relatively objective measure, the severity of headaches and the urgency of the need for professional help are, of course, more subjective. In the end, you must judge for yourself how profoundly your headaches are interfering with the quality of your life and whether you will take the time to care for them properly. However, because of the progressive nature of chronic headache, it may not be easy to achieve an honest perspective on your situation. Feedback from others who are close enough to you to be honest can be invaluable. Try to be open to those who care enough to tell you what they see. Don't kill the messenger (an old saying, but a wise one). The following questions also might help you consider how things are.

1. Are you using more and more medications while your headaches remain just as (or become even more) frequent?
2. Have you started taking medication even before you have a headache, for fear that one might develop?
3. Are you missing time with your family because you just have to get to bed when you come home from work?
4. Do you notice dissatisfaction or disappointment from family or friends because you had to miss yet another outing?

5. Have you been making excuses to avoid social commitments for fear you would have a headache while you are out?
6. Are you missing work more frequently, with some threatening comments from your boss?
7. Are you avoiding long trips for fear they will be interrupted by headaches?
8. Do you sense skepticism from your doctor about the amount of medicine you must ask for?
9. Have you found yourself crying unexpectedly and without obvious reasons?
10. Do you seem to be functioning less sharply?
11. Do you become acutely fearful at early signs of pain?
12. Have you been more irritable than usual?
13. Are you beginning to have headaches almost every morning?
14. Have you noticed soreness and stiffness of your neck and shoulders, with more headaches?
15. Is it hard for you to tell why headaches come on? Do they seem to have a "mind of their own"?
16. Does it seem as if you just have pain all the time?

If you answered yes to even a few of these questions, you have a severe and chronic headache problem; you really owe it to yourself to get competent professional help from a headache specialist. Most of you already will have consulted a physician; few people have this much pain without at least trying to find help. But many of you will not have had good luck in this effort. Chances are that you are reading this book because the help you've received is not enough at this point, as the following case illustrates.[1]

✦   WHEN SIMPLE TREATMENT IS NOT ENOUGH: THE CASE OF BETTY S., PART 1

Betty S. was twenty-nine when she had her first severe headache. She had experienced occasional headaches in the past, but most of the time she could take mild painkillers and get rid of them quickly. Then one day she felt the pain not only in her head but also in her neck; it was so intense that she felt nauseous. The acetaminophen that usually took care of the pain made no noticeable difference, and

---

[1]All cases in this book are composites. No resemblance to any individual is intended.

the headache continued for hours. Finally she went to bed. It took a while, but she eventually fell asleep. When she awoke the next day, she felt tired and groggy, but the headache was gone. Her worry lingered, but thoughts of calling her doctor vanished as she hurried to get ready for an important conference. *What caused that awful pain?* she wondered on her way to the office. *I hope that never happens again.*

In fact Betty had no severe headaches until three months later. She had almost forgotten about the first one. But this time the headache returned in force; it seemed even stronger, forcing her to leave the restaurant where she and her husband had met for dinner. She noticed she could feel it in her left ear and in her jaw too. The next day Betty made an appointment with her primary care physician, who examined her thoroughly and ran a series of tests. The results were negative, and Betty's physician could find no sign of underlying disease. He suspected the headaches might have been the type called migraine but was not yet sure; he prescribed two pain-killing medications, one an analgesic compound with codeine to be used with severe headache and one aspirinlike drug called a *nonsteroidal anti-inflammatory (NSAI)* for less severe pain. He asked Betty to call the next time she had a headache to report how she did with these medicines.

Betty soon began to notice that she had less severe headaches more often than she thought. Most of the time they went away with the NSAI medication. Her next severe headache occurred two months later, but she used the painkiller with codeine as instructed and stopped the pain before it ruined her weekend. These results seemed positive, and her doctor advised her just to call if she noticed any change in the severity, frequency, or character of the headaches. For the next year Betty's headache pattern remained about the same, and she became accustomed to using her medications when needed; sometimes she increased the dosage or decreased the interval between doses when the pain refused to subside.

As Betty turned thirty, she noticed that her severe headaches were coming closer and closer together. She also found that her "garden-variety" headaches were more frequent as well. Soon she was having some type of headache almost every other day; Betty began to feel almost like a victim in response to them, as if they were some malevolent presence that came and went as they pleased, invading her life without a clear pattern.

Betty's doctor tried to help. He changed her prescription several times, but nothing seemed to work for long. He sent her to a neurologist for an examination and more extensive tests, but again no disease was discovered. Betty was taking over-the-counter painkillers along with her prescription drugs, eventually using some kind of medication nearly every day. Betty's doctor was almost as frustrated by her problem as she was. Here was a patient who was now calling several times a week, sometimes from the local emergency room, and who he knew was taking more medication than was healthy, despite his many warnings against it. And her symptoms were, if anything, getting worse. He had tried to broach the subject of a psychologist, but Betty stiffened in response and evaded the whole issue. She had agreed to see a physical therapist but, she told the therapist, just didn't "have the time" to devote to a long-term program. Out of desperation Betty began to grasp at any advice she could get—from friends, newspaper articles, TV documentaries— and she consulted an ophthalmologist and an allergist on her own. Nothing helped.

Finally, when she was thirty-three, Betty came to our university's headache clinic. Betty's case and several others like it had moved her doctor to attend a lecture given by one of the authors, and after some consultation he referred her to us. As she told her story in the first session, she realized that it seemed like a long time ago that it had all begun.

HOW TO FIND HELP

Betty S. was fortunate. Though it took some time, she did (as we relate in Chapter 2) ultimately receive the multimodal therapy that made her headaches manageable and her life enjoyable. The big step that made a difference for her was finding her way to a headache specialty clinic. Her family physician had done everything he could to manage her pain. As in most cases, his diagnostic workup had been competent and the choice of medications reasonable. However, when the headache did not subside, Betty and her physician were caught in a bind. She began to use more medication and began to manage her own care, seeking out specialists in various areas. Her life was organized around her headaches. Her physician made efforts to refer her to appropriate specialists and thought even of using a psychologist and a physical therapist. His patient's reluctance to commit to such treatment and her desire to resolve the problem "simply" (primarily with medicines) made it more difficult for him to get her into a comprehensive headache clinic.

The Comprehensive Headache Clinic

If you and your primary care physician are unable to find a solution for control of your headaches, it is time to consider seeking an opinion from a comprehensive headache clinic. If your physician has not suggested such a referral, no insult is implied in asking him or her about the idea. Most primary care physicians will feel quite comfortable in dealing with this question and in helping you find a reliable clinic. Physicians are trained to recognize the areas in which they and their patients would benefit from consultation with a specialist. They will also be able to use their professional organizations and contacts to find a headache clinic in your area that has a staff of varied professionals who can carry out multimodal treatment. The comprehensive clinic directs care in the area of headache only, leaving the primary relationship with the family physician intact. Information about treatment, with the permission of the patient, is passed along to the family physician's office.

If your doctor does not bring up referring you to a headache specialist, you might say something like, "Doctor, you know we have been working with these headaches for some time. They really are still very frequent, even though I know you are doing your best. They are causing me distress in my life, and I would like to have a different perspective on their management. I understand that you have examined me [or referred me for examination] to rule out serious disease as a cause of headache, so I am not too worried about that. However, I would like to have a thorough review of my headache history and medical status to see what factors might be keeping this headache going and what we might do about it. What do you think?"

While some physicians in solo practice specialize in headaches, most often the kind of multimodal (often called *multidisciplinary*) treatment we are discussing in this book will be found in a clinic setting, either free-standing or associated with a university or large medical center.

A comprehensive headache treatment center is usually staffed by a variety of health professionals who work together to provide multimodal headache treatment. Various levels of care are available. While outpatient treatment is the most common way to care for the headache patient, inpatient units are usually available to handle people in intolerable pain or severe emotional distress and those in need of intensive medical or behavioral treatment. Outpatient care may take the form of regular office visits or an organized program often called a *day hospital.* In the day hospital the patient lives at home or in a hotel or other accommodations arranged through the clinic.

These are the professionals you are likely to meet in a comprehensive headache clinic:

Physicians

The most common types of physician in comprehensive headache clinics are neurologists and internists. You will also find psychiatrists, physicians who specialize in human behavior. When working in a headache clinic, they are trained to work not only with mental illness but also with the emotional factors that affect headache. Physicians hold an M.D. or a D.O. degree. The common link among all physicians in a specialty clinic is their interest in difficult headache problems and their desire to apply the knowledge of their specialty to the resolution of headache problems.

Psychologists

Psychologists specializing in headaches have received special training to apply principles of human behavior to the management of headaches. This will range from using special techniques like biofeedback to affect physical events leading to headaches to managing the emotional distress that typically comes with headache. They will be licensed to practice by a state board, just as physicians are. A psychologist typically will hold a doctorate, with the designation Ph.D. or Psy.D.

Therapists

Two other important professionals in comprehensive headache clinics are physical therapists and biobehavioral therapists. Physical therapists are trained to work with the effects of muscles on headaches. They deal with the effects of chronic muscle tension or poor postures that often aggravate chronic headache. Biobehavioral therapists help to carry out the treatment plan developed by the psychologist or psychiatrist. They use behavioral techniques and psychological therapies to help control physical events that lead to a headache or make it worse. They often implement the biofeedback techniques.

Nurses

Nurses are a very important part of any headache team, filling a variety of responsible roles, depending on the center. They typically work with physicians at every step of the diagnostic and treatment process and at every level of care. They may be your first professional contact at the clinic and may handle your calls when something is not going as planned.

✦

At any clinic you may find other professionals as well. If you encounter any professional designation or title that is unfamiliar to you, don't hesitate to ask for clarification of that person's role on your team.

In this book, when we say *doctor* we mean physician, psychiatrist, or psychologist. If it's important which one, we will specify. When we say *therapist* we mean a professional working under the direction of a doctor to help patients carry out their treatment.

Comprehensive headache clinics are not made with a cookie cutter. Each will be different, reflecting the perspectives of its founding or current team. Some headache clinics are heavily oriented toward diagnosis and medication; most are more comprehensive in the treatments they commonly use. An initial workup at the more comprehensive headache clinics will include two perspectives: the medical and the psychological. A typical evaluation will include a series of medical visits with the physician and nursing team, including any necessary tests to rule out disease. Your prior medical records will ordinarily be requested to give the physician a background on your health and to avoid unnecessary duplication of any tests.

The psychological evaluation is different from what you might expect. Many people worry that a psychologist is looking only for evidence of serious mental illness. It *is* necessary to screen for mental illness, but the great majority of people coming to comprehensive headache clinics do not have such problems. The psychological interview concentrates on a thorough history of your headaches, seeking details that will help pinpoint emotional or other factors that bring on or aggravate your headaches. In addition, the psychologist wants to determine how you learn best, with the idea of helping you develop new skills for headache management. In general, the psychologist is there to help you gain as much control as you realistically can have over your headaches and to help you become a fully participating member of the treatment team. Details of the multimodal diagnosis and treatment process are given in Chapter 2.

As you can see, many people are involved in a multimodal treatment process. If your headaches can be managed safely and effectively with medication only, you will surely choose that route. However, if they are not responding to such treatment, a comprehensive headache clinic is for you. You can also see that, although in theory multimodal care can be provided by a solo practitioner with a network of affiliated professionals, it is more difficult to achieve coordination of care if all the professionals are not part of the same group. Communication is essential to the multimodal treatment process. It is difficult under the best of circumstances, but extremely difficult when practitioners are spread out in a variety of independent offices across a metropolitan area. Remember the last time you or someone you know chose to act as his or her own contractor on an addition to the home or some other large job? Communication under these circumstances requires more time than most busy private practitioners can afford.

Ideally, then, the primary care physician remains at the center of your overall care, supplying your medical records to the headache clinic and then staying informed by the clinic, with your permission, of your diagnosis, treatment, and outcome. The headache clinic issues a final report once your active care is completed, and your doctor carries on with the remaining medicines, referring back to the clinic if you have a relapse.

Finding a Comprehensive Headache Clinic

If you find yourself in the position of having to locate a headache specialist on your own, try the following sources:

- ✦ National Headache Foundation, (800)843-2256
- ✦ American Council for Headache Education, (800)255-2243
- ✦ Authors of headache treatment articles in professional journals: ask your local librarian for help
- ✦ Local university hospitals, often a good source of knowledgeable physicians and psychologists who direct or can refer you to a specialty clinic

Both the National Headache Foundation and the American Council for Headache Education sponsor support groups in various locations around the country and offer reliable sources of information, including newsletters.

Ask First

When checking out a particular treatment center, ask questions. It is important to be assured that you will be taken seriously and that the evaluation process will be given sufficient time to ensure that your headache problem is understood in detail. In multimodal treatment your participation is critical; you are a real part of the treatment team. You should expect your questions to be answered directly, even if part of the answer is, "We don't know yet." Your observations and ideas are also important, and you should expect not to be patronized or dismissed offhandedly when you have a theory about your own headaches. You may not be right, but you are capable of understanding the reasons for not following up on an idea or how an idea is checked out scientifically. There is no reason that you cannot become an expert on your own chronic headache.

This kind of involvement in the treatment team is, of course, a double-edged sword. It requires a level of commitment that not everyone relishes. Truthfully, most of us just want to be "fixed" when we have a medical problem. While this is perfectly normal and understandable, if you have a chronic and severe headache problem that is not responding to medication alone, you may be better off taking on this level of responsibility in the treatment of your headaches.

Here are some questions you may want to pose before making a decision regarding a headache clinic. You might also reflect on them while in the early stages of treatment.

+ How much time is given to making the diagnosis?
+ How much time will be given to hearing your headache history?
+ How long is the typical course of treatment?
+ What fees are charged and how? How are insurance, HMO, and PPO arrangements handled?
+ What types of professionals are part of the standard workup?
+ What types of professionals are available for specialized consultation?

- ✦ Whom can I call when I have questions, and how long will it be before my calls are returned?
- ✦ If I have problems during treatment, is someone on call twenty-four hours a day?
- ✦ How will I be kept informed regarding initial impressions, assessment of my progress, and reasons for using or not using various diagnostic procedures and treatments?
- ✦ What types of treatments are most commonly used? Is this a clinic with one treatment that is used for all, or is the treatment plan designed flexibly to reflect my particular situation?

WORKING TOGETHER

As you'll learn in more detail in the next chapter, control of chronic headache is the mutual responsibility of doctor and patient, who can be seen as the co-captains of the treatment team. The unique nature of headaches imposes unique requirements on both parties. The doctor must respect the patient's report of pain and his or her observations regarding the pattern of headaches and the effect of treatment; the patient must accept the responsibility for carrying out the plan flexibly and be open to all possible factors affecting headaches, including his or her own thoughts, behaviors, and feelings.

Too often we see that patients whose headaches are not easy to control end up feeling that no one cares; they interpret the frustration of their physician as demeaning or uncaring. Too often physicians feel trapped between an escalating headache problem and patients who push for more medicine and/or will not consider behavioral treatment for fear of being considered "psych" cases. We often cajole our own patients with the idea that they can choose whether or not to "use their head," but they can't choose to eliminate its role in their headaches. We suggest to our physician colleagues in primary care that the most satisfied chronic pain patients will be those who are treated not only with knowledge but with respect, understanding, and empathy. For the chronic headache patient a comment such as "The problem is all in your head" should never be more than a statement of the obvious.

WHAT YOU SHOULD EXPECT
FROM YOUR DOCTOR

Any professional who is going to treat you for chronic headache should also be a person you feel comfortable with. The following are some characteristics that often contribute to a positive doctor–patient relationship. They are essential qualities in a comprehensive headache clinic. You have a right to expect such characteristics in the person to whom you are entrusting so much.

Your doctor should:

+ Demonstrate genuine care for you and interest in your problem.
+ Be a good communicator, educating patiently and understandably.
+ Be able to discuss psychological factors without giving you the message that your pain is not "real."
+ Be flexible and listen attentively to your questions and observations.
+ Adjust the treatment plan to reflect new information.
+ Not answer every increase in headache only with new or more medication.
+ Work patiently with you even when the headache does not lend itself to a quick solution.
+ Be willing to consider multiple factors contributing to the same headache problem.
+ Be ready and able to coordinate efforts with all other members of the treatment team, including you.
+ Include you in goal setting.
+ *Take time*—to listen to you, to follow through on coordination of treatment, to give you feedback, to educate you.

WHAT YOUR TREATMENT TEAM
WILL EXPECT FROM YOU

Multimodal therapy for chronic headache is both empowering and demanding. You play a crucial role in the treatment process. Nothing done *to* you is going to control your headaches; only what is done *with*

(cont.)

WHAT YOUR TREATMENT TEAM
WILL EXPECT FROM YOU *(cont.)*

and *by* you will have a positive effect. If you're not prepared to meet the demands of this role, you will lose out on the considerable rewards of taking this approach to treatment.

You as patient should:

+ Be prepared, as anyone else with a chronic illness, to participate actively in managing your disorder.
+ Become knowledgeable about your own condition, using books and tapes recommended by the team.
+ Not wait passively to be "cured" of your headache through the ministrations of others.
+ Be open to a variety of treatment options in addition to medication. Recognize the value in nonpharmacological therapies, including lifestyle changes as necessary.
+ Not press your doctor to come up with more and more esoteric, invasive, or otherwise risky therapies to avoid effort on your part to deal with headache.
+ Follow the plan your treatment team comes up with (using the checklists in Appendix I to keep track of your participation in treatment and its effects). Try to work with their suggestions and bring ideas for modifying the plan back to the professional who developed it with you. (There are two ways to really sink a comprehensive treatment plan: do nothing the team asks of you, or do everything they ask of you exactly as they have written it—nothing more.)
+ Take the time to keep records, practice the techniques, observe changes in your body, identify headache triggers, and respond appropriately, as you've learned, to early signs of headaches (again, use the checklists in Appendix I to record your efforts and observations).
+ Be open to the role of psychological factors. Let go of the stereotypical idea that the psychologist is there to determine whether or not you are sane or your headaches are "real." Recognize that psychological factors along with physiological factors almost invariably play a role in persistent headache.

✦

CHAPTER 2

Consider Your Options: The Multimodal Approach

Headache, as explained in Chapter 1, is essentially a chronic illness. Like diabetes, chronic headache cannot be cured, but it can be managed effectively. When it is managed well, there are relatively fewer headaches. When it is managed poorly, the headaches are frequent and disabling. Management of a chronic illness means attending to all the factors that contribute to the problem—such as eating habits in diabetes and, as we shall see, psychological stress in headaches.

As you may know from personal experience, however, some headache problems are difficult to manage. People come to our clinic after they've tried a variety of over-the-counter and prescription medicines and a sometimes bewildering array of self-help techniques picked up from friends, family, and media. No matter how competent their prior treatment has been, the fact is it hasn't reached its goal. From the time these people make the first call to our clinic, we know the odds are that no simple answer to their problem will emerge; if there were one, their family physician already would have found it.

In our opinion, the optimal answer for people with this type of headache problem is multidisciplinary evaluation and multimodal treatment. At our clinic and at an increasing number of others throughout the United States, behavioral and physical therapies are emphasized as much as medication in the treatment plan. Usually the several types of treatment are employed simultaneously, each addressing part of the problem. Evaluation is ongoing through the treatment process, and we consider many possible factors that might be affecting the individual headache problem.

Successful multimodal treatment also requires an element that cannot be supplied by any of the professionals available at a headache clinic: self-management. As Chapter 1 mentioned, *you* are a crucial member of your own treatment team. If multimodal treatment is to succeed in helping you control your headaches, you must be invested in learning about headaches, committed to identifying and recording the pattern of your headaches, and dedicated to "hanging in there" as you and your treatment team work away at your problem. Patient and team must agree not to give up on each other. Flexibility is certainly a requirement, as is consulting professionals outside the clinic as needed, but perseverance above all is the basis of the contract between patient and team.

When we left Betty S. in Chapter 1, nothing her doctor had tried to do for her was working, which brought her to us.

✦ TAKING CONTROL OF HEADACHES: THE CASE OF BETTY S., PART 2

When Betty came to our clinic, she was having severe headaches several times a month, most often on the left side and including pain in the jaw, ear, and neck. On the worst days she also had intolerance for noise, painful sensitivity to light, nausea, and even vomiting. A typical severe headache for Betty lasted at least six to eight hours but might linger until the next day. Ascribing any pattern to the headaches had become more and more difficult, but they did seem to occur more often on waking and especially on weekends. She also had less severe headaches almost every day, with pain in the forehead or the back of her head.

Betty's initial workup with us involved a physician's and a psychologist's evaluation. The former revealed that she was taking medications for high blood pressure, backache, nasal congestion and inflammation, fungal infection, and estrogen replacement. The latter revealed that her severe headaches had started at around the time she and her husband had moved from their longtime residence to a smaller house. Conversation with both of them revealed that Betty was remarkably aware of how her headaches in the past could be brought on by emotional upset, by drinking red wine, or by eating citrus fruits. However, as her headaches became more frequent, it had become more difficult for her to make any sense of why they started.

She felt her headaches seemed to come as they wished and experienced them almost as if a foreign invader were taking her over.

Betty's doctors recognized her severe headaches as a type of migraine. Because they were so frequent, it was necessary to emphasize prophylactic (preventive) medication instead of abortive medication or painkillers. As we will see later, taking the latter type of medication too frequently can actually make the problem worse. Betty was instructed to take regular doses of a medication called a *tricyclic antidepressant* that would work to reduce the frequency and severity of her headaches, improve sleep, and boost mood. Her doctors did not expect this medicine to solve the problem entirely. She also needed to withdraw from the regular and frequent use of the other medicines she had been taking for headaches. Further, they urged her to improve her general health as much as possible—for example, quitting smoking and reducing fat in her diet. They recommended a regular aerobic exercise program as part of the comprehensive program but recognized that she would have to start with very gentle exercises like walking to avoid aggravating her difficult headache condition. In addition, they recommended consultation with a specialist in sinus disease and allergies who was known to the clinic team, to get a reliable diagnosis of her nasal congestion.

Betty's doctors felt that stiffness of certain neck, upper back, and facial muscles was probably aggravating her headaches, including her less severe ones, which they called *tension-type headaches*. They asked the physical therapist to see her for a more detailed assessment and to work directly on these muscle groups in an active, exercise-based program.

After the psychologist's evaluation, the team also asked the biobehavioral therapist to take Betty through the behavioral plan for managing headaches. This plan included keeping careful track of the headache in a diary that recorded several factors that might be related to her headache. The team realized that she was probably correct in not seeing any pattern now, since the headache was so frequent. However, they explained that as the headaches became less frequent her skill in observation would be a valuable tool in identifying triggers in her particular headache. Betty was told also that the team was not looking for a single cause of headaches but the pattern of triggers that increased the likelihood of headache on any given day. In addition, the biobehavioral therapist would teach Betty how to relax more fully, using biofeedback equipment to help her learn accurately and efficiently, to use this relaxation in realistic life situations, and to notice more quickly the early signs of headache so that she could respond with medication, muscle relaxation, and overall calming.

In addition to these general plans for the behavioral treatment of headache, Betty told her psychologist about specific sources of stress in her home and work life. She enjoyed her job in an accounting office but found one co-worker difficult, as did others working there. In her effort to be kind, Betty was the only one in the office who would eat lunch with this person. She felt pressured both because she did not really enjoy these lunches and because she felt deprived of this period of relaxation with her other co-workers.

Betty's husband had recently lost his job. He was increasingly irritable, and she felt that trying to avoid upsetting him was like "walking on eggshells." She felt even more pressure to maintain her own job performance and was frustrated by his apparent unwillingness to help more around the house while he was unemployed. She was also busy caring for her father, whose second wife had died not long before. She visited her father's home every night. The psychologist felt that the psychological stress brought on by these home and work situations probably contributed to Betty's everyday headaches. Betty needed to find a way to spend a little less time tending to others and a little more time on herself, without ignoring her sense of responsibility to work and family. The psychologist would ask the biobehavioral therapist to help Betty find ways to evaluate her own needs as well as those of others, to be more assertive with family, and to use available social resources for help.

Betty's progress to date has been good. She hasn't been able to follow through on all the advice of her health professionals, but what she has done has been quite successful. First, Betty stopped her previous regimen of pain medication and started taking the tricyclic antidepressant. She was given additional medication to use when she had severe headaches, but with strict limitations on its use. Second, Betty went to physical therapy sessions to work primarily on her neck muscles. She also kept a total of twelve appointments with a biobehavioral therapist over about six months. At first she went weekly, but gradually she tapered her visits to every other week and then to every month. With the biobehavioral therapist Betty practiced relaxation of her whole body and used biofeedback equipment to learn to maintain relaxation of important muscle groups that were being addressed in physical therapy, especially in the course of a normal day. She practiced relaxation at home and still does brief relaxation exercises at work. This also helped Betty become more alert for early signs of the muscle tension that was one way stress was triggering her headaches. Betty and her therapist developed options and strategies for change in her home and work situations.

With the help of her biobehavioral therapist Betty worked out reasonable ways to decline some invitations to lunch by her unpopular co-worker. She has started socializing more with other co-workers in the office. At home Betty told her father she would visit him three nights per week and began to work with him to reconnect with old friends. She also had a little good luck: her husband found a new job.

In this process Betty had to follow through on some very difficult decisions and learn new skills. At first some of these new behaviors seemed quite awkward, even selfish. Her therapist could help her sort through these feelings, but Betty had to make the decisions—and, most important, act on them.

Betty's headaches? She's had migraines less than once a month—instead of about once a week—since she started on this plan of treatment. And though she still gets mild headaches at work, they are less frequent and she is able to stop them by using relaxation techniques and making limited use of painkillers.

HOW MULTIMODAL THERAPY WORKS

A mode is a way of looking at something or a way of going about something. As you'll see throughout this book, both of these meanings apply to the work of the comprehensive headache clinic team—and to what we want to help you do for yourself—with headaches. In the initial and ongoing evaluation of headaches your team looks at a headache problem from a number of perspectives: Is your headache a part of your biological heritage? Is it related to a disease or some other organic condition? What other factors seem to be making you susceptible to headache? From among these many perspectives your team hopes to single out the ones that seem to offer the best return on your efforts to take effective action against the problem. These will be factors that have overriding importance in triggering headaches or that affect multiple other factors interactively. In our example Betty S. learned to look at her headache from multiple perspectives—as a medical problem, a muscular problem, and a stress problem. This helped her cooperate with the team in attacking the problem from several directions at once—by means of medication, muscle relaxation, and reduction of stress.

We believe that in the case of chronic severe headache not only is there more than one way to take control, but in most cases using a combination of ways at the same time—a multimodal approach—will be more effective than using any one of those ways in isolation. Had Betty S. continued with medication alone, ignoring muscle tension and stress, she probably would not have found the remarkable decrease in her headaches, and there would have been greater risk of temporary or minimal improvement.

Betty S.'s case illustrates some of the more common ways headache sufferers can regain control: (1) modifying the type of medication and the way it is used in the treatment plan, (2) addressing the important area of muscle irritation in chronic headache, (3) recognizing early signs of headache and responding to them effectively, (4) improving overall health habits, and (5) reducing sources of stress in everyday life by learning new skills and changing perspectives on difficult situations. Betty got the best prescription medication for her headaches and reduced her overall intake of painkillers and abortive medicine. She learned and used relaxation techniques. She took actions that, while in themselves no doubt stressful, led to an overall decrease in everyday stress.

In Chapters 6–9 we will discuss in more detail the different therapies in a multimodal approach. Here it's important to understand two points about the broad-based plan for treating headaches. First, overuse of painkillers and abortive medications actually seem to increase the risk of more frequent pain among headache patients. In the worst situations, overreliance on medication can lead a patient into a vicious circle: more frequent headache requiring more medication leading to more frequent headache and so on. (Chapter 6 discusses so-called rebound headache in more depth.) A multimodal approach to headache management, combining appropriate medications with the range of nonmedication treatments, increases the odds that the patient can break this cycle for the long run.

Second, medication and nonmedication approaches to treatment are all addressing the same end—the physical events that together make up the biological event we call a headache. It is a mistake to think of some treatments in a multimodal plan as affecting the body and the others affecting the mind. It is only the method and the mechanisms that vary among treatments; all are designed to affect physical function. What we call mind, body, and spirit are all part of the same individual system. When your team uses biofeedback equipment to teach relaxation to reduce the effects of psychological stress, the goal is to change a behavior that changes the body. Throughout the treatment process there are many such examples of the interplay between psychological and physical events.

For that reason we give the psychological or behavioral parts of treatment the general heading of *biobehavioral therapy.* The therapists who carry out many of the psychologist's recommendations are called *biobehavioral therapists,* a category of professionals introduced in Chapter 1. Biobehavioral medicine—*bio* for biological and *behavioral* for what people do and how they act—to put it simply, describes those parts of treatment that use behavioral or psychological methods to affect physical functions. Biobehavioral therapies are part of behavioral medicine and are effective strategies in the treatment of disorders with significant psychological and biological aspects that are inseparable in evaluation and treatment. The end result is a more integral, more holistic approach, and this approach defines *multimodal* as we use it in our practice. Understood in their broadest sense, all disorders have psychological and physical elements, but this model has been most important in advancing treatment in chronic disorders such as headaches.

WHAT YOU CAN EXPECT AT A COMPREHENSIVE HEADACHE CLINIC

No two clinics are exactly alike, but a description of the process followed in our own program will give you a reasonably good idea of what you might encounter at most comprehensive headache clinics.

After you have made an appointment and prior to the first evaluation interview, you will be asked to complete a questionnaire regarding your headache history, current headaches, medical history, personal history, and current health habits. In addition, if there is time, you will be asked to begin completing a headache diary. The diary gets you started on what will be a critical part of any biobehavioral treatment you might undertake. Not only does it give your team information, but it also makes you a better observer. Most patients find that, unless they prepare by completing the questionnaire and diary, even what should be very familiar information may be hard to recall during the first visit in a new office.

It is also very easy to forget to bring up important information unless you write it down beforehand.

Medical records are necessary. You will be asked to authorize the release of medical records from anyone who has seen you for headaches in the past and from your primary care physician(s). These records give the team a "leg up" in understanding your history and the nature of your headaches. They also may eliminate the need for some types of medical tests or suggest the need for others.

All these different forms of preliminary information serve as different forms of memory: the questionnaire is your current recollection, the diary is a type of "current" memory written day by day, and, medical records are an external source, written by someone else at the time those events were happening. You may also have some type of personal record that you have saved—you may, for example, already have used the checklists in Appendix I on your own—which will also be valuable to you and the team.

The initial evaluations will include, at a minimum, interviews with the physician and psychologist. There will also be a physical examination. On the basis of the data gleaned, the physician will inform you of any tests that are required. These might include x-rays, blood work, magnetic resonance imaging (MRI), and a computed tomography (CT) scan. Additional consultations may be scheduled to identify or rule out possible contributing factors such as allergy, sinus disease, temporomandibular dysfunctions (TMD), or any other disease or problem the initial workup may suggest.

A great deal of time in these first interviews and in the review of medical records is given to obtaining a detailed headache history. The psychological review includes as well an assessment of your current emotional state, the impact of the headache on your sense of well-being and on your ability to function in normal home and work roles, the meaning of this pain in light of your life experience to date, your usual methods for coping with pain, your optimal learning style (especially important for the interactive biobehavioral therapy), and the state of your current home and work environments.

Other information that will be requested in the course of the initial evaluations will have to do with the state of your muscles and with health-related lifestyle. Posture, muscle tenderness, and range of motion are important indicators of potential problems with the muscles that may affect headaches. The most important areas for this examination are the upper back and shoulders, neck, and face (especially the muscles used for chewing). You may be asked to sit, stand, or move in certain ways or to remain passive while the physician tests your joint areas and presses into some of your muscles. As we discuss in Chapter 4, exercise, diet, sleep, alcohol, tobacco, and caffeine are important lifestyle factors in many headache problems. If your physician or psychologist spots a possible problem in any of these areas, he or she may ask more detailed questions.

During these first visits it is important that you ask all the questions that occur to you and that you share any information you think might be important. Don't hold back information because you want to see if the professionals on your team will come up with it themselves. Do ask if you are worried about the possibility of a specific or serious disease; put aside embarrassment, ask the question, and listen to the answer. Most of the time it will relieve you greatly. If you're uncertain about the reason for any evaluation, the results of tests, or the reasoning guiding the workup, let your team clarify for you. At the end of the evaluation, ask for a clear description of the next steps in treatment. It is important to everyone that you understand so that you can participate actively in your own care. However, it is also easy for any member of the team to slip into using technical language or jargon or to rush through an explanation in the course of a busy day.

This initial evaluation might be squeezed into a few days or extended over a period of several weeks, depending on the clinic schedule and your availability. It may sound like a complicated process, but in practice it is carried out flexibly. The personal relationships between patient and individual members of the team go a long way toward making the evaluation less stressful and more supportive.

The treatment plan will flow from this evaluation process. When everyone is communicating well, the resulting plan should make sense to all involved, including you. However, on any given day, clear communication may be a tall order. When the plan does not seem to make sense, it means only that you and the team must review it to see if it needs to be changed or explained further. The most common components of a treatment plan for chronic severe headache are changes in medication, physical therapy, and biobehavioral therapy. In any given plan, depending on need, any number of other components may be included, but not for every person.

The frequency of behavioral therapy visits is individualized, but the most common interval is weekly. The content of biobehavioral therapy is also individualized but commonly includes working with the headache diary, enhancing education, using biofeedback to assist in relaxation training or specific muscle relaxation, and learning to monitor signs of a headache or physical signs of stress early enough to do something about them. The therapist will help you build a greater understanding of your particular headache pattern based on your actual experiences and observations, feed back this information to the doctors, lead you in practicing activities suggested by the doctors, and otherwise help you make the general treatment plan work for you.

Your physical therapist, building on the information obtained in the initial evaluations, will make a more detailed assessment of your muscles. Based on this assessment, the therapist will recommend exercises for stretching and strengthening and may use other methods like heat, electrical stimulation, or massage to help your muscles relax. Physical therapists also look at structure and movement, which would include your various postures and gait.

Keep in mind that this entire process will vary depending on the headache center you visit. Each clinic will have a different emphasis in evaluation and treatment. The common characteristics of a comprehensive headache clinic are the ability of different health professionals to work together and the willingness of the staff to use a variety of evaluation and treatment methods, selected to fit your particular case. If the clinician seems to offer the same type of treatment to all the patients who come to the clinic, you are probably not in a comprehensive headache clinic.

HOW MUCH IMPROVEMENT CAN YOU EXPECT?

The outcome you can expect from your investment in multimodal treatment varies. So much depends on an effective patient-treatment team collaboration. It is important to remember as well that headache is not cured but managed. Outcomes reflect the extent to which headache frequency, intensity, and duration are reduced.

There are few studies of the outcome of multimodal treatment (by any name) in actual headache clinics. Most studies have focused on certain types of treatments compared to no real treatment or other types of treatment. Many have been done in research settings rather than in comprehensive headache clinics. Informal data available for our clinics and others indicate that 50 to 65 percent of the patients who participate in treatment do very well with multimodal treatment in the headache clinic. Only 6 to 15 percent indicate that they receive very little or no benefit from care.

The reasons for failure to benefit are many. In some cases the patient and treatment team did their best but to no avail. In other cases the patient simply did not like the kind of treatment offered. Not all patients are receptive to the idea of learning to work with their own headaches. Some see only medical or surgical options as "real" treatment. These people tend to vote with their feet: they either do not participate in the behavioral part of treatment or leave early in the treatment process.

In short, our clinical experience and that of others suggests that there is every reason to expect success in managing your headache if you are willing to be open to the multimodal model of evaluation and treatment and if you will give yourself to the effort. Genuinely trying to follow the recommendations of your treatment team and helping the team modify its plan to fit your particular situation more and more closely increases the likelihood of your controlling your headaches. The checklists in Appendix I can help you keep track of how closely you're adhering to your treatment plan and any changes in your headaches over time. Perhaps just as important, though, are your motivation and expectations. Both unrealistically high and despairingly low expectations seem to produce less success or outright failure. Both can interfere with your ability or willingness to work hard, as part of the team.

Follow-up care is another important point. Since we have said already many times that the headache problem is not cured, it follows that in one sense treatment must be continued indefinitely. It may be discouraging to hear this, but the situation is no different from taking medication for high blood pressure; if you stop, it is likely that your blood pressure will rise again. The good news is that the most active phase of treatment may last only about two to three months. When a patient comes to a comprehensive clinic from some distance, the first part of treatment, inpatient or intensive outpatient treatment, is done over a period of weeks at the clinic, with additional outpatient therapy scheduled closer to home. Biobehavioral therapy visits usually extend beyond the most active phase, with biweekly and then monthly visits for the next several months. Preventive medications are usually kept up for a longer period, but eventually they too are withdrawn. After the period of active treatment, paying reasonable attention to positive health habits, managing stress levels, and catching early signs of headaches should be all that is needed to keep headaches under control. As Betty S. illustrates, usually you can expect to maintain long-term control with just small changes in attitude and lifestyle.

As with any chronic condition, you may have relapses, but that does not mean the treatment didn't work in the first place. You do need to call one of your doctors to review what has happened and to confirm the diagnosis. If you can put your finger on the reason for the relapse, you will be able to get control again quickly and will have learned something to prevent relapses in the future.

✦

CHAPTER 3

Know Your Symptoms: Major Headache Groups

Oone of the first things most people with headaches want when they visit a headache clinic is an explanation for their symptoms: "Why am I having this kind of pain?" "Why isn't it going away as it used to?" This process of diagnosis is the first stage for the professional team as well. Initially the team tries to determine what the headache *is not*. Ruling out the serious diseases that have headaches as a symptom is always a concern, for professional and patient alike. Worry that the headache is the result of a brain tumor, for example, is not unusual. Fortunately, it is also rare to find such disease.

When medical examination and specific tests have failed to produce evidence of disease, the team begins to focus on what the headache *is*. Now the headache itself becomes the primary focus, and its various symptoms are categorized using rules published by the International Headache Society. The clinician goes further, trying to work with you to identify the specific mechanisms by which your headaches are produced and the specific factors that trigger them. The categorization of headaches and the identification of mechanisms and triggers gives the professional team valuable information regarding treatments that are likely to be helpful and gives you direction as you try to find a pattern in the confusing experience of frequent pain.

In describing some of the more common types of headaches, this chapter is not meant as a substitute for a professional diagnosis. Only a professional can ask the questions that lead to an accurate diagnosis and explain the particular headache pattern you're experiencing. The general *categories* that we describe here are the most common, but there are many others that may be important in your particular case. The *mechanisms* of headache can be described in general, but a description that will do justice to your particular situation must be so precise as to be beyond the scope of this book. We can discuss the theory behind identifying *triggers* of headaches and note the more common ones, but your particular array must be uncovered individually, hopefully by someone who has the experience to recognize not only the most common but all possible triggers.

Multimodal evaluation and treatment are based on the premise that headache is a complex syndrome. Even when the headache types are identified, there is an intricate web of contributing factors and triggers that set headache in motion. Evaluation must be directed toward uncovering all risk factors and pinpointing those that are most potent. Only then can your treatment team begin to work on eliminating them.

The treatment tailored uniquely for you will be a product of both the type or types of headache you have and the specific factors that are triggering the headaches. This chapter addresses the more common types of headaches; Chapters 4 and 5 discuss triggers.

THE LIMITATIONS OF LABELS

Before we get into the major headache classifications, a few more words of caution: Putting a name to your headache is important, but it is only a first step. Remember again that chronic headache cannot be cured, only managed. With frequent severe headaches the odds are always against your physician's being able to identify one particular medication based on your headache type that will cure the problem. No matter which type your doctor determines that you have, in fact, your part in headache management will remain largely the same. It is that cooperative effort that much of this book is directed at and on which we suggest that you concentrate.

As noted earlier, the professional diagnosis will be specific to you, with a detailed evaluation of mechanisms and triggers. There are many different types and subtypes of headaches and many more factors that have been identified as headache triggers for at least some people. Addressing all the possible combinations is beyond the power of a single book. Even the most comprehensive textbook cannot do justice to the individual; none of us have seen a textbook description come to life and walk into our offices. You may have a more unusual type of headache or more than one type. You may be one of the very few with a particular trigger. If you have frequent severe headaches, especially chronic daily headache, you may have difficulty recognizing any particular headache subtype or trigger in yourself because it is very hard to see beyond the near-daily experience of head pain and its associated malaise. So it is important not to assign yourself the diagnostician's role when you read this chapter. All the considerations that go into a professional diagnosis must be addressed in the individual clinical case and observed over time with an open-minded professional who can help you sort fact from fallacy.

For these reasons the review of headache types in this book will not be detailed or exhaustive. Here we provide an overview of salient points about some of the most common types, points that may be especially relevant to your understanding of and participation in treatment.

LOCAL HEAD OR NECK PAIN

As we use it in this book, *local head or neck pain* is a general term meaning pain that does not fit one of the typical headache categories but is bothersome enough to bring people to a headache clinic. It usually originates from irritation of a muscle and its surrounding tissue, commonly called *soft tissue irritation or injury,* but it may also result from irritation of the bony structure—a joint or the spine of the neck.

Depending on which muscles or joints are irritated, special names may be assigned to your particular type of local pain. Cervicogenic (originating from the neck) headache is one such type. Temporo-mandibular dysfunctions (with their various subtypes), discussed in Chapter 10, might also be described as a type of local pain from the perspective of the headache specialist.

Local in the term *local head and neck pain* means the pain occurs in a limited area, most commonly the occiput (the back of the head), one temple, the side of the head, or the cheekbones. The pain is more often steady and dull rather than sharp or throbbing. It may get worse with use of the affected muscle or joint, and the muscle or joint often feels tender when pressed. Remember also that if the local irritation sets in motion a pattern of pain recognizable as one of the common headache types, that category will be used to describe your headaches.

TABLE 1. Major Headache Groups

	Local head and neck pain	Tension-type headache	Migraine headache	Cluster headache
Onset of headache	Gradual	Gradual	Attack	Attack
Location of pain	One place, often occiput or cheekbone	Broader "band" around head	One or both sides, one or both temples	Behind eyeball
Type of pain	Steady or shooting, mild to moderate	Dull, mild to moderate	Moderate to severe, pulsating	Severe, drilling or boring
Duration of headache	Minutes to days, until source of irritation is relieved	Hours to days	Four hours to several days	One-quarter hour to several hours

Irritation of the muscle or joint may be caused by an accident or by subtle and persistent overuse. The latter can occur even if the stress on the muscle does not seem severe in itself. For example, poor posture may place extra demand on neck muscles, or clenching the teeth may put pressure on jaw muscles. In some cases certain postures also weaken a muscle from underuse, making it vulnerable to irritation from very mild activity.

These kinds of muscle or joint irritations can occur any number of times in your life. In most cases local head or neck pain is treated by addressing the source of the pain, and the pain subsides as the irritation of the muscle or joint is eased. Usually the problem is resolved quickly with rest, medications, and gradual return to activity. However, when the pain does not respond in a timely way, local head or neck pain can be a candidate for multimodal therapy of the type described here. If you consult a comprehensive clinic for persistent pain of this type, your treatment team may prescribe physical therapy in conjunction with biobehavioral therapy (behavioral therapy often including the use of biofeedback) to soothe the muscles, restore muscles and joints to optimal functioning, increase your awareness of the postures you tend to adopt, and teach you how to relax the targeted muscles. Chapters 7 and 8 go into detail on physical therapy and relaxation techniques.

TENSION-TYPE HEADACHE

Tension-type headache is the most common of headache complaints. In this type of headache a dull pain spreads across a larger area of the head than with local head or neck pain. It is typically felt on both sides of the head as opposed to the often one-sided nature of local pain. Many people describe it as feeling like a tight band around the skull or like a cap on the top of the head. It may be accompanied by mild sensitivity to light or noise, blurred vision, light-headedness, and a general sense of not being "with it." Some scientists think of this type of headache as a less severe relative of migraine, and in fact there is some overlap of symptoms between the two, although they appear in milder form in tension-type headaches.

When this common headache occurs infrequently, it is usually treated with analgesics (painkillers). Many people report that such headaches occur when they are stressed, and they may use them as a signal to slow down or take a break. But when tension headaches begin to occur more frequently, there are many pitfalls, including the risk of analgesic overuse and analgesic-induced or rebound headache (see Chapter 6 for details). Tension-type headache can develop into one of the subtypes of chronic daily headache, a near-daily experience of this dull pain that wears you down slowly but steadily.

At one time tension-type headaches were known as *muscle contraction headaches,* so called because it was believed that muscle tension, or excessive contraction, was the sole cause. Certainly tension-type headache can be triggered by muscle tension of the upper back, neck, or face, but this type of headache can also occur without muscle tension. Again, the overlap between symptoms of tension-type and migraine headaches has led some clinical specialists and researchers to suggest that they are related rather than completely distinct headache types.

For these reasons multimodal therapy in a headache clinic can be the indicated treatment for tension-type headaches. As the headaches become more frequent, a number of triggers and other contributing factors may come into play. Muscle irritation may suggest the use of physical therapy and biobehavioral therapy in combination. Biobehavioral therapy may also be used to help track down less obvious triggers and to help you identify early signs of a headache so that you can respond before it gets out of hand. This will help you reduce your reliance on painkillers to control the headache. The persistence of chronic tension-type headache may lead your physician to prescribe preventive medication in addition to the analgesics (see Chapter 6).

MIGRAINE HEADACHE

Migraine is the best-known and most-studied type of severe headache. Among those beyond the age of puberty, migraine affects twice as many women as men. It's not certain exactly how many suffer from migraine, but among young adults the prevalence has been estimated at about 30 percent for women and 17 percent for men. These figures decline as age increases. Unlike local or tension-type headaches, which build more slowly to peak intensity, a typical migraine is more like an attack of pain—there is a clearer beginning, a period of peak severity, and then a tapering off, with the whole attack (unless modified by medications) lasting from four hours to more than one day.

The most common image of migraine is a headache that occurs on only one side of the head, at the temple. The word *migraine* derives originally from *hemikrania*, Greek for "half the skull." The fact is, though, that migraines can cause pain on both sides as well as on one side of the head. You may feel the pain at the temples, but you may also feel it at the front or back of the head. Typically the pain is accompanied by nausea and vomiting and moderate to extreme sensitivity to light and noise. On average the pain is more intense than from tension-type headaches, and you may have difficulty carrying out mildly exerting activities such as climbing stairs. Those with untreated or inadequately treated migraine often must take to bed, trying to sleep, until the attack passes.

Your doctors will need to consider the many subtypes of migraine in evaluating your problem. One of the more dramatic subtypes is migraine with aura. Often occurring thirty to forty-five minutes before the onset of pain, aura may consist of a single symptom or a combination of symptoms. Because they last only a short time and seem to originate in the brain, these symptoms are known as *transient neurological symptoms*. The most common are visual symptoms such as wavy or jagged lines in one side of your field of vision, blind spots in one or both eyes, or flashing lights. Some auras take nonvisual forms as well: disturbance of smell, numbness, tingling, or paralysis on one side of the face.

Although aura is a dramatic and possibly frightening experience, only a small minority of headache sufferers experience it. You should also understand that aura is distinct from the more general headache prodromes—less specific and more subtle symptoms that may precede the onset of a headache and indicate either increased or decreased physical arousal. Examples of prodromal symptoms are increased appetite, heightened sensitivity to light or noise, high energy or fatigue, irritability, and a sense of not being sharp. Prodromal sensations may precede headache with or without aura by several hours or longer and are useful as early warning signs of a headache. While they are more difficult to notice and link to headaches than aura, prodromal sensations often allow you even more time to act to abort a headache.

Migraine is sometimes called *vascular headache* because it is associated with constriction (narrowing) and then dilation (expansion) of blood vessels at the temple. However, it has become evident that this is not the whole story in migraine. For one thing, dilation alone does not necessarily cause pain. For example, when we exercise, our vessels dilate, but that usually doesn't cause a headache. The vascular dilation present in migraine is now more often understood as part of the final phase in a complex series of events originating in the brain and leading to a headache.

As with tension headaches, migraine may be triggered by a large number of factors. At one time a laundry list of names was given to identify migraine headaches triggered by specific factors. Now it is generally agreed that migraine should be identified by its symptoms, as outlined briefly here, rather than by the factors that may trigger it in a particular case. As we will see in Chapter 4, there are many possible triggers of migraine, but few *always* cause migraine, even in any one person, and very few, if any, cause migraine in all individuals. Tracking down the relevant factors triggering headache can be frustrating since it is often a matter of working with probabilities rather than uncovering the "smoking gun" or single cause.

When a migraine attack ends, it is said to be in *remission*. During remission there are no migraine attacks—but this is not necessarily a period of no headache. As was the case with Betty S., most migraine sufferers also have tension-type headaches in between the migraine attacks, another reason many specialists think of these two headaches as related. The tension headaches may seem inconsequential in comparison to the migraines, but tackling them is an important part of multimodal treatment of migraine. They may be said to form part of the ground from which more frequent migraines may arise. Frequent tension-type headaches also increase the risk of analgesic overuse.

In the case of migraine headaches, your physician will seek an effective abortive medication for you. Given the very severe nature of migraine pain, abortive medication is crucial to eliminate hours of unnecessary suffering. This type of medication, when taken promptly, can cut off the migraine headache before it runs its course and hopefully before it reaches its peak intensity. For frequent migraine headaches, more than two per month, many specialists will want to consider preventive medication as well, since overuse of abortive medications may prolong your headaches and contribute to the development of chronic daily headache. The headache specialist in a comprehensive headache clinic will also want to take advantage of the nonmedication treatments for the same reasons; see Chapters 7–9.

CLUSTER HEADACHE

Cluster headaches are so named because they occur in bunches or clusters with periods of no headache in between. They are much less common than migraine, estimated at less than 1 percent of the population according to most experts. They are found in men much more often than in women, with the ratio estimated at five or six to one. Each cluster is a series of regularly occurring headaches, usually relatively close together. It is not unusual for such headaches to occur at the same time of day or night each day when a cluster is in process. The individual headaches may last for from half an hour to several hours. The duration of clusters varies widely but may last for months; the period of remission that follows also varies in length but can extend even to years.

The interruption of sleep and the sense of powerlessness that you may feel when a cluster headache starts at night is part of the toll of this type of headache. But it is the severe localized pain that is most vexing; it is described as intolerable. Sufferers usually feel the pain around and behind one eye and often describe it as "boring" or like a nail being driven into the eye. A number of symptoms, on the same side of the head as the pain, can be associated with cluster headache, including drooping eyelid, tearing from the eye, bloodshot eye, and running nostril.

Although cluster headaches occur mostly in men, new syndromes similar to cluster headache that occur in women are now being described in the medical literature, though they are thought to be rarer than cluster headaches. The pain is similar to that reported with cluster headaches but lasts for briefer periods of time that occur more frequently. These syndromes often have been found to be responsive to a particular type of nonsteroidal anti-inflammatory medication called *indomethacin.*

Fortunately, most cluster headaches can be treated successfully with medication. Some medications are prescribed to abort the individual cluster headache; others are used to abort the entire cluster period. However, there is a chronic form of cluster headache as well. Respites between clusters may grow shorter; in severe cases they may disappear altogether. In such chronic cases a modified form of multimodal therapy may help. Preventive medication is often prescribed. To augment medication, a headache specialist might suggest biobehavioral therapy to help the patient cope more effectively with the pain and to reduce factors that seem to be associated with increased risk for or exacerbation of the headaches (see Chapter 4). However, there seems to be less experience with multimodal therapy for this type of headache than with other forms of headache.

CHRONIC DAILY HEADACHE

Chronic daily headache, described in Chapter 1, affects an unknown number of people. Very little information has been amassed, but one study found that about 5 percent reported daily or near-daily headache.

Chronic daily headache can be divided into subtypes, but they are not always easy to define in any individual. Chronic tension-type headache is one type, but many of those with chronic daily headache also report having migraine symptoms on some headache days. Among these people, many started out having recognizable migraine headaches, with tension-type headaches between attacks, but progressed gradually to what seems to be a mixture of tension-type and migraine headaches that are difficult to describe in isolation from each other. As you'll learn in Chapter 6, one of the most common reasons for the development of mixed headaches is overuse of analgesics and other medications. However, some people do seem to develop such headaches after accidents or otherwise without medication overuse.

Chronic daily headache can be difficult to treat. Even in cases where the intensity is not severe, the fact that the pain is ongoing can erode your energy and sense of well-being. It can become debilitating, seriously undermining your satisfaction in work, family, and friendships. Depression is not an infrequent result. Overuse of analgesic medication makes treatment an uphill battle; other medications that might be helpful and nonmedication treatments seem to be made less effective.

Efforts to treat chronic daily headache by attacking one facet of the problem—adding a new medication, resolving depression, or relieving muscle irritation, to give three examples—are often frustratingly ineffective. People with this type of headache sooner or later find their way to a comprehensive headache clinic. They come saying they have tried "everything" to get rid of their headaches. Fortunately, most headache specialists have much experience in assessing such problems and designing multimodal solutions. Evaluation depends on what we have seen are the hallmarks of the comprehensive headache clinic—consideration of all possible factors affecting headache and use of multiple modes of treatment to address the most potent of these factors. Nonmedication treatments play important roles in these multimodal treatment plans, allowing medication to do its job without leading you to rely too heavily on that part of treatment.

◆

Obviously, a great deal more could be said about each of these headaches and about those headache types not included in this chapter. For additional detail, see "Further Reading" at the back of this book. Keep in mind, too, that membership in the National Headache Foundation or in ACHE comes with a subscription to the excellent newsletters published by these organizations, rich sources of ongoing information on many aspects of headache evaluation and treatment.

✦

CHAPTER 4

Causes and Triggers of Headaches: An Overview

"Take more time for yourself."
"You've got to learn to relax."
"Don't worry so much."

Chances are you've heard this kind of advice more than once. Your physician has ruled out disease as the cause of your headaches. You and your doctor also may have made valiant efforts to identify causes of your headaches and to eliminate them one at a time. Yet your problem has improved only temporarily or continues unabated, and the question "Why do I have these headaches?" remains largely unanswered.

It is a sensitive subject with many people who have headaches, but your doctor probably is on the right track in implying that that modern-day tyrant, stress, is playing a role in your headaches. Psychological pressures are typically found to be the most common trigger of chronic severe headache problems. In fact we hope that this book will discourage you from thinking of psychology and medicine as "either . . . or" approaches to understanding and treating headaches. To unravel all that is behind your headache problem, you need both physicians and psychologists on your team.

On the other hand, the relationship of psychological factors to headaches is complex. Their presence certainly does not imply that your headache pain is not real. Psychological stress results as much from the almost-constant headache pain as from anything else. So your doctor also was correct to investigate a number of other possible factors. As this chapter will explain, most often several factors are at the root of chronic headache. They can be of many different types, including but not limited to psychological stress. They operate at the same time, interacting with each other. For that reason it is seldom profitable to try to eliminate such factors one at a time.

Finally, your doctor's advice to relax and unburden yourself is on target as well. Successful management of headaches often relies on relaxation—physical, emotional, mental, and spiritual. But generalized prescriptions such as the ones that open this chapter are obviously too vague to be much help. That's where the other professionals available to you at a headache clinic come into play—the therapists and biobehavioral specialists who can show you how to achieve true relaxation and implement other lifestyle changes that will work with your medication to get your headaches under control.

The aim of this chapter is to give you an understanding of the mechanisms by which various factors cause or contribute to chronic headaches. Chapter 5 focuses on your role in working with your doctors to identify the specific factors that affect you.

First, definitions of a few terms:

Symptom versus Syndrome

To define your headache as a certain type (see Chapter 3), your headache team has to know as much as possible about your experience with the headache. Your physician first tries to determine if there is any specific disease of which headaches are a *symptom*. If no such disease can be found, the focus of evaluation and treatment shifts to the symptoms themselves. Chronic headache of this type is considered a *syndrome,* a collection of symptoms without a known, curable cause. The headache itself is named on the basis of the symptoms it includes.

When headaches cannot be identified as a symptom of a known disease, it is no longer possible to hope for cure. However, we do know effective ways of treating the syndrome—ways we will explore in more detail in the chapters that follow. Treatment is focused on alleviation of the symptoms themselves and elimination or modification of the factors that lead to them. This treatment is of necessity multifaceted. Specific interventions are added to the treatment plan based on the symptoms and factors targeted as most bothersome or powerful. Our focus in this book is on chronic headache as a syndrome—and what you can do to reduce its frequency, intensity, and duration.

Internal Tension and Psychosocial Factors

In this chapter you'll encounter two important causes that involve your psychological state and the way in which your psychological state affects your body. One is *internal tension,* the buildup of stress by your body. The other is *psychosocial habits,* the way you think about yourself and interact with your friends, family, and co-workers. Understanding internal tension and psychosocial habits is a necessary prelude to important non-drug therapies discussed later in this book.

Headache Factors

When we say that most headaches involve a number of factors, what, exactly, do we mean? The term *factors* may refer to anything that leads to a headache or makes it worse.

A huge number of potential factors can affect headache activity, including but not limited to social events, thinking patterns, emotions, foods, environmental changes, certain ways of taking medication, muscle tension, and internal tension. If you can work with a doctor or therapist to identify major factors affecting the frequency, intensity, or duration of your headaches, you've taken an important step toward developing an effective treatment. This part of treatment will consist of finding ways for you to avoid such factors, reduce their impact, or at least be prepared for them so they don't catch you by surprise.

Triggers and Contributing Factors

The factors involved in your headaches can be classified according to how they affect you. The *early signs* of a headache, whatever sets it off, are critical to notice. These signs may be actual beginnings of the headache or physical events that almost invariably lead to a headache. Catching the very early signs of a headache, perhaps even before pain begins but certainly before it becomes severe, can give you an important leg up on controlling headache. These early signs may be prodromal symptoms, symptoms of aura (both discussed in Chapter 3), aching muscles, cold hands, a general sense of tension, or any number of other indications. As you learn to observe your individual headache pattern more closely, you will begin to notice these indicators. As you become more confident in dealing with them, you will view them as an occasion for effective action rather than dismay. We call this ability to notice and respond to early signs of headache *somatic awareness.*

A factor is a *trigger* if a headache regularly occurs within a short time after it is present. If you drink red wine, do you usually have a headache within a few hours? If so, we would call red wine a trigger for you. Or if you often get a headache after eating sharp cheese, we would call the cheese a trigger.

Those examples are, however, oversimplified. In actuality most people's headaches are triggered not by one factor at a time but by the interaction of several. For example, chocolate may set off a headache if you are otherwise upset and tired, but it may have no apparent effect if you eat a small amount when you are otherwise relaxed. In general, the more triggers that are present at any given time, the more likely a headache is to follow. Although for you one specific trigger may be so powerful that you have a headache whenever it appears, the effect of most of your triggers is a matter of probabilities. This interaction among triggers is what confuses and discourages so many people seeking a pattern to their headaches. It is not uncommon for us to hear a patient say, "I thought that [one specific factor] caused my headaches, but now I am not so sure."

In one study migraine patients reported an average of five triggers. This has important ramifications for the way we treat headaches. It demands that triggers be observed systematically over time and that all of the most likely candidates be considered. We do this by focusing on (1) triggers derived from research on headaches that list the triggers many people have reported and (2) hypotheses generated from your own experience. We ask you to record headache activity, physical sensations, and potential triggers in a diary. Then, when a specific factor seems to be important, we set up small experiments in which that factor is purposefully eliminated or included so we can see the effects. This kind of comprehensive effort is much more likely to be effective than simply trying to cut out one factor at a time, and it is not as hard as it might seem if you have experienced helpers to guide you.

It's important to emphasize again that classification of factors as triggers depends ultimately on how they operate in you. We simply do not know enough to tell you ahead of time exactly what factors will trigger headaches in you. What is a trigger for someone else may not be for you, and vice-versa. We start with general information from the collective experience of headache specialists regarding likely triggers, but we end with a profile of your particular and unique experience. That kind of individual attention is where success lies in headache management, and it is the reason that in this book we so strongly emphasize the *process* of headache management and working with a headache clinic to get control of your chronic severe headache problem.

Factors that increase your vulnerability to headache but don't immediately lead to headaches in themselves we call *contributing* or *contextual factors*. Such factors create a context in which a headache is more likely to be set off by triggers. If you are constantly under stress, never exercise, get insufficient sleep, have irregular sleep hours, emphasize animal fats in your diet, eat irregularly, eat too much or too little, smoke tobacco, or drink very little water, your lifestyle is making it more difficult to prevent headaches. Additional factors, such as alcohol, caffeine, and analgesic or abortive medications, have the potential to be *addictive*. These factors make headaches more likely as they are used up in your body and require more of the same to stop the headache.

As you can see from this partial list, we are really talking about habits of self-care. In our experience, the healthier your lifestyle, the more successful you will be in managing your headaches.

✦ THE CASE OF KAREN L., PART 1

Karen was thirty-nine when she came to us, a single mother with three children. She had been divorced ten years before. She attended college and worked part-time. Karen had headaches every day, with pain beginning in the back of the head and neck and spreading to the temples, more often on the left side than the right. She wasn't aware of any pattern in their duration or any particular factors that might be associated with them. Recently she had begun to experience a new type of pain—a burning in the right top of the head.

Karen was referred to our clinic by a neurologist, who had diagnosed her as having chronic daily headache, a combination of migraine and tension-type headaches. The neurologist had tested her reflexes and ordered MRI and CT scans, which revealed no neurological damage. The neurologist also had prescribed an antidepressant and an analgesic compound, advising her to discontinue using another painkilling drug that she had received from her primary care physician.

When she came to the clinic, Karen reported to our doctors that in addition to the antidepressant and analgesic prescribed by the neurologist, she was using medicine from another doctor to clear chronic sinus congestion; over-the-counter analgesics, which she took frequently and on her own; and an estrogen supplement, prescribed by her gynecologist following her hysterectomy five years earlier. She was also using the analgesic compound more frequently than suggested by her neurologist; she was surprised to find, when she completed her diary, that she was using at least one nearly every day. Medication itself, our doctors concluded, might be a factor in Karen's headaches (more on this subject in Chapter 6).

We then worked out a detailed history of Karen's headaches with help from a questionnaire and a detailed interview with one of the psychologists specializing in headaches. As far as Karen knew, there was no history of headaches in her family, but she was not sure about the health history of her maternal grandmother. She recalled that her headaches had begun after puberty, while she was in junior high school. By the time she finished high school, they were occurring three or four times a year and were quite severe, lasting two or three days. As Karen described them, these headaches sounded like migraines. At that time there seemed to be no connection to her menstrual cycle. Starting about four years before coming to the headache clinic, Karen began to experience less severe headaches in between her migraine headaches. These new headaches were more frequent than the migraines and seemed to fit the description of tension-type headaches. Over the last year she noticed that both the migraine and tension-type headaches had become progressively more frequent. By the time she came for help, she was having headaches more than twenty days per month on average, and it was becoming harder to tell the tension-type and migraine headaches apart. This information supported the neurologist's diagnosis of chronic daily headache.

The physical examinations identified significant muscle tenderness at the upper back and jaw, particularly on the left side. The muscles at both temples were tender. When they tested her range of motion, the doctors found that Karen could move her neck normally but that movement caused some pain at the back of the neck on the left side. Her mouth opened fully and without pain, but Karen herself was aware that she often clenched her teeth. Based on this information, the doctors recommended physical therapy to lessen Karen's muscle tension. We will describe this part of her treatment more fully in Chapter 7.

Karen had been married right out of high school and divorced eleven years later. Despite some counseling, the divorce had been bitter, with much conflict over custody of the children. In the past two years things had improved somewhat. Still, Karen told the doctors that she felt nervous, "really stuck" in her situation of trying to manage a four-person household, work, and go to school at the same time. She had difficulty relaxing because she felt guilty about taking a break when there was so much to do. Although she had been socially active in high school and during her marriage, she didn't have time for much social life now. Karen said she thought about her situation a lot but came up with only "lots of problems with no answers." She conveyed a general sense of discouragement and disappointment.

This psychosocial review led Karen's psychologist to suspect that she suffered from mild to moderate depression. Her doctors also found that she thought herself too busy to bother with exercise or regular mealtimes. She slept for six hours each night and was often sleepy during the day. She drank lots of caffeinated soda but not much water. While Karen didn't drink much alcohol, she was a two-packs-a-day smoker.

The recommendations we made for Karen's treatment are described in Chapter 5. For now, her case illustrates clearly the many factors that can be present in chronic severe headache. Medication overuse, muscle tension, internal tension, psychological and social strains, and poor health habits—the factors described in more detail in the next section—all seemed to have a potential bearing on Karen's headaches.

THE MAJOR FACTORS IN HEADACHES

In the broadest sense, taking control, for Karen and other headache sufferers, requires an attitude of reasonable self-regulation. With a chronic disease like headache, you cannot control everything. You can't control the fact that you have headaches in the first place. There is nothing "fair" about it, but now you have to manage your health and the factors that lead to headaches more closely than does a person without chronic headache. The story is the same as for diabetes and many other chronic illnesses: chronic headache is a biological disorder, but behavioral factors, including psychological stress, are very important in its management.

The good news is that a great deal can be done to reduce the number of headaches you have, how long they last, and even how painful they become. If you can work with this general attitude, accepting the facts you cannot control and working with the factors you can influence, you will do much better in taking control of your headaches. Because many factors typically come into play and interact with each other, a comprehensive approach to management that takes into account as many of these factors simultaneously as is practical is usually most effective.

Predisposition to Headaches

Migraine and tension-type headaches seem to run in families. The research in this area gives us some reason to think that migraine headaches, in particular, may be genetically inherited. In addition, sharing the same family "environment" may increase the likelihood of your having headaches. So it is fair to say that if you have chronic severe headache you have probably come by it "honestly." Most likely you were born with or received at an early age the propensity to have these headaches. This is not something you can choose.

On the other hand, it does not mean everyone in a family will have migraine. You may be the only one in the known family history who has severe headaches, and you may have brothers or sisters who have never known what a severe headache feels like. It does mean that if one of your parents or grandparents—or even aunts or uncles—had chronic headaches, you may be more likely to develop them, too. If an unusual variant of headaches runs in your family, it is also wise to let your treatment team know about it; what is true for your relatives may be true of your headaches as well.

Disease

Many medical conditions can have headaches as a symptom, and this is why your physician's initial investigations focus on disease as a possible cause of your pain. If an underlying disease is found, it can be treated and the headache relieved. Because the causes of headache are many, the initial diagnostic workup is critical. However, specific and curable disease as a cause of chronic and recurrent headache is rare.

Most people reading this book will already have seen their primary care physician, and many will have been referred to a neurologist and other specialists to try to rule out disease as a cause of the headache. When the diagnostic search reaches the point of rapidly diminishing returns, it makes sense to begin treating the headache as a syndrome and to look for the more usual factors affecting headache frequency. Of course, it is very important that you continue to monitor the headache activity with your physician and report any new symptoms or unusually severe headache pain. Now the search turns to the model of multiple and interacting factors affecting headache as well as factors resulting from the reaction to headache that make it worse or better. In other words, at that point the multimodal approach to controlling your headaches, from diagnosis through treatment, is likely to be the more effective.

The Menstrual Cycle

There is no doubt that headaches in women are more common around the time of menstrual flow. In some cases women will have their only severe headaches at this time. The headache seems to occur most often before flow, but there may be regular headache during or after flow or even associated with ovulation. Migraine associated with menstruation is especially problematic. This is not the same thing as premenstrual syndrome, a condition that must be diagnosed by specific criteria more extensive than headaches associated with the menstrual cycle.

The association with menstrual flow seems to arise from the fluctuations in hormonal levels, especially estrogen, rather than from too much or too little of any particular hormone. There are other associations of headaches with hormonal changes. Many women trace the onset of their severe headaches to near puberty. Headache is often, but not always, worsened by birth control pills. It is common for migraines to ease or disappear altogether in the second and third trimesters of pregnancy. Care must be taken in selecting hormonal supplements after menopause; some types or some schedules of administration may increase headaches. The relationship between hormonal levels and headaches is complex, and it is difficult to say anything that will be true for all women. What is safe to say is that this is an important area that must be considered carefully in the multimodal evaluation and treatment plan.

Medication

The same might be said of your medication. Medication is a critical part of any treatment plan for headache. However, with chronic headache it is important not to expect medication to do the whole job. It is this reliance on medication-only treatment that can lead to more troubles than you started with. In some cases medications taken for chronic headache may end up actually aggravating or intensifying headaches (see Chapter 6).

As a rule of thumb, the more you can simplify your medication regimen and reduce overall medication intake, while still getting good control of headache, the better for you and for your overall effort to take control of headaches. This rule applies especially to analgesics, or pain-killers.

Muscle Tension

Almost all individuals with chronic headache have some degree of muscle irritation at the upper body—the upper back, the neck, and the face. The muscle irritation is most often associated with chronic but subtle muscle tension, nothing very dramatic but going on regularly day after day. This is as true (or truer) for migraine headache as for tension-type. Muscle irritation should be considered a trigger of headache pain. The type of pain triggered reflects a variety of factors, not the least of which is the type of headache to which you are prone. Muscle irritation can produce local pain, pain around the site of the muscle irritation, or it can refer pain to sites away from the irritated muscle. For example, muscle irritation at the back of the neck may be felt as severe pain at the temple on the same side of the head. This would be called *referred pain* and is one of the reasons for cervicogenic headache—pain at the front and side of the head that originates from the neck. Finally, muscle irritation can trigger any of the major headache types we have discussed previously.

Chronic muscle tension may arise from a variety of causes—regular poor posture, repeated muscle strain or overuse, tightening up under stress, muscle habits or mannerisms such as frowning or grinding the teeth, or even bracing against headache pain itself. Over time this tension may lead to very tender muscles, aching with normal movement, stiffness from being in one position for a long time, pain when you lie in bed for very long, or even restrictions in the extent to which you can move your neck or jaw.

Health Habits

The frequency and intensity of your headaches can be affected by exercise, sleep, environment, and diet. Poor choices in these areas lead to a general decline in health and greater susceptibility to headaches, and they also can be specific triggers of headaches. A 1992 article on headache triggers in *Headache Quarterly* reported that in recent surveys of headache patients of various nationalities "one-third to one-half . . . believe stress, alcohol, environmental extremes of temperature, light or sound, biorhythm irregularity in sleep or eating, and certain foods all have induced some of their headaches." As we have noted before, the fact that you are prone to have headaches is no reflection of your character or even your lifestyle; however, the responsibility to manage factors like lifestyle that can affect how often or how long you have headaches falls very much on your shoulders. You have not chosen to have headaches, but you are making choices now that will affect how much they interfere with your life.

Smoking

By now public-health crusades have made the debilitating effects of smoking on overall health well known. If you suffer from chronic headache, you may have one more good reason for quitting. Smoking seems to be a negative factor among those with chronic pain conditions in general. It is commonly believed to be an important aggravating factor in cluster headaches in particular. The way in which smoking tobacco might be associated with exacerbation of pain conditions is not known with certainty, but there are many possible routes, and none of them are good for your health.

Exercise

Lack of regular physical exercise can leave you more susceptible to chronic headaches, and regular exercise can actually reduce your risk. Several points are critical in making effective use of exercise. First, do it regularly but not severely. Prevention of pain depends on regular aerobic exercise, not on becoming an Olympic-class athlete. Walking is an excellent aerobic exercise and can frequently be done with others to get the added benefit of social support. Second, use stretching exercises as part of any regimen. Maintaining flexibility is a good way of avoiding injury or strain. Third, slow down or stop if you have increased pain from your exercise. Ask for advice from a professional on types of aerobic exercise that will not aggravate your pain. Fourth, always start a new exercise program under the general direction of your physician and let him or her know if there are any worrisome symptoms when you start. A regular exercise program will leave you feeling better in many ways.

Sleep

Sufficient, regular, and good-quality sleep is very important to your sense of emotional well-being and very important in regulating chronic headache. Unfortunately, sleep is one of the first casualties as headaches strike more frequently. It is not unusual for those with severe and frequent headaches to have trouble getting to sleep, to wake with pain during the night, and to feel in the morning as if they have hardly rested. This may be associated with the headache syndrome itself, but it may also reflect improper use of medications, caffeine, or other substances that affect sleep. When depression builds, a common fact in chronic headache, sleep is disrupted further, even to the point of waking in the wee hours of the morning and not being able to get back to sleep. The tension of stressful lives also takes its toll on the quality of sleep, leading to restlessness and to unrecognized sources of muscle tension like grinding the teeth while sleeping.

Your first goal should be to establish regular sleep hours. Too much sleep or irregular sleeping or waking times can be as much a problem as too little sleep. Sleep postures are also important, though difficult to control. Sleeping on your stomach puts a strain on your neck muscles. Poor pillow arrangements or mattresses that give inadequate support may irritate muscles by placing them in awkward positions for long periods of time. If you have regular difficulty with getting to sleep or staying asleep, be sure to discuss this with your treatment team. There are safe medical and behavioral treatments for evaluating and changing these patterns.

Environment

In this day and age, we are certainly all aware that our environment has an impact on our health. When we talk about chronic headache, however, *environment* means more than the general conditions of our world. Headache risk can be increased by many environmental factors over which you have no immediate control. Although we may think first of problematic conditions such as air quality in the home or workplace, and these should certainly be considered, headaches are affected more often by climatic environmental conditions such as weather changes or seasonal changes that increase natural allergens such as pollen or mold counts.

For most people who have found weather changes associated with headaches, the risk increases when rainy weather approaches. These conditions are more often found in the spring and fall. Others find that headaches are worse in summer, when hot and humid conditions may prevail.

Allergens, which can increase headache risk, may arise not only from changes in the plant cycle but also from commonly occurring factors in the home: pet dander, dust, tobacco smoke, fumes from paint and cleaning products, or molds in furnace ducts or houseplant soils. Allergy is rarely the only cause of headaches, but it may act as a trigger. It should be suspected when there are other obvious symptoms of allergic reaction, and the diagnosis should be made or ruled out by a competent specialist. If there is chronic congestion as well, sinus infection, acute or chronic, should be ruled out.

Among the many other factors in your environment that might be considered, be sure you are comfortable with the intensity and type of lighting available for any given task. Dim or glaring lighting in your home or work area may lead you to squint or otherwise strain the muscles around your eyes. Seating and work surface arrangements also are often designed poorly, exacting a toll on muscles of the upper back and neck. Even crowding and noise levels may increase tension or arousal, leaving you more susceptible to headaches.

Diet

Diet affects headaches in both general and specific ways. Generally, eating regularly—a small meal or nutritious snack every three to four hours—keeps blood sugar levels relatively stable. Also, following the kind of diet recommended for general good health—low in fat and high in vegetables, fruits, and grains—seems to reduce headache risk. Whether there is a causative relationship or whether diet affects headache sufferers differently from other people we cannot say, but we see many headache sufferers who don't eat well. They may consume too much caffeine or alcohol, fat, sugar, or salt or too little water, complex carbohydrates (whole grains, beans), fruits, and vegetables.

For some people certain foods are specific headache triggers. These foods set off headaches directly, usually within hours of ingesting them. There is a great deal of information on dietary triggers of headaches.

Entire chapters and even books have been written for headache patients on foods to avoid. However, it is a difficult area in which to give specific advice that applies to everyone. Few foods affect every individual. In many people a given food will trigger headaches, but not every time or under all conditions. Even less can be said with certainty about the particular mechanisms by which foods cause headaches.

We do know that some foods show up very frequently as causes of headaches. Some common examples are red wine, aged cheeses, yellow cheeses, processed meats (for example, ham, bacon, hot dogs, or salami), foods with monosodium glutamate, and dark chocolate. Many other foods show up as triggers less frequently but have been documented in at least some reasonable proportion of patients.

Diet is a more complicated factor to sort out than you might think from a casual review of headache self-help information. Certainly there is no reliable test to determine food allergies, and some people have ended up needlessly on very restrictive and complicated diets without affecting headaches very much. A general list of foods to avoid is not much better; many of these foods will not affect you, and some foods not on any list may be your nemesis. What is required is a system for researching the role of dietary triggers in your particular situation. More information on a system to do just that is given in Chapter 5.

Internal Tension

Internal tension is our name for your body's response to stress. Most common sources of stress in our lives reflect the interaction of circumstances with our interpretation of and response to them. Whenever we perceive ourselves as potentially overmatched, overwhelmed, or otherwise threatened by circumstances, our bodies release hormones and other chemicals that affect many systems, including heart rate, breathing rate and volume, blood flow, muscle tension, digestion, mood, and mental awareness. The stress response rouses us for "fight or flight." Usually, as the perceived threat lessens, the body relaxes again. A certain degree of internal tension is appropriate for any given situation; without it, we could not respond to the ever-changing demands placed on us in our lives.

However, internal tension can become a contextual or trigger factor in headache. If you are very vulnerable to headaches, whether by the biological propensity itself or by the combination of other trigger factors present at any given time, normal arousal can in itself set off headache.

Frustratingly, this arousal may be associated even with a pleasant event. One of the curses of the child with migraine, for example, is a headache on the occasion of a birthday party or a special outing.

In another frustrating pattern, a prolonged period of arousal can be followed by a headache, just when everything seemed to be getting back to normal. For example, weekend headaches can be associated with relaxation after a difficult week. It is also not unusual for headaches to become worse *after* doing relatively well during the difficult time of caring for a sick relative or working out the details of a funeral and burial.

Some people have, in addition to the propensity toward headache, an extreme physical response to stress. Sometimes they are called *hot reactors*. The physical responses may be combined with recognizable emotional reactions such as anger or anxiety. When this pattern is combined with a propensity for headache, the impact of the stress response as a trigger of headaches is much magnified.

Internal tension also may build gradually over time. Some people seem less able to let go of worrisome thoughts, unsettling emotions, or stress-increasing behaviors. Do you tend to worry about things over which you have no control, dwell on how others perceive you, feel too responsible, feel helpless, set high (almost unattainable) standards, feel controlled by deadlines and time pressures, or deny problems rather than confront them? Do you hold on to emotions such as anxiety, fear, guilt, anger, or depression or brood over hurts? Do you hold anger in to "keep the peace" rather than assertively defining and resolving conflicts? Do you allow yourself to get too busy, conform always to the schedules of others, work excessive hours, or neglect to set aside time for yourself? These are some of the common behaviors that, when done repeatedly, become a style of living leading to depression and chronic stress. They can trigger specific headache episodes and create a fertile breeding ground for chronic headache in general.

Psychosocial Habits

Earlier we discussed the kinds of behavior we usually associate with health, the physical health habits of sleeping, eating, and exercising. Equally important are the psychological and social (psychosocial) health habits, those involving our patterns of thought, feeling, and relationship with others. We can't see, hear, taste, touch, or smell these, but we know that our sense of well-being is affected by them—so are our overall health and our headaches.

Just as we make choices in the tangible areas of our lives, we make choices in the intangible areas, and these choices have important implications for us. Over time, these choices become habits, our psychosocial health habits. They become customary ways of viewing the world in which we live, positively or negatively. Joy in what is and optimism in what will be are traits to be cultivated, not just gifts you have either received or not. So often we go through our daily lives practically asleep, acting as if everything is happening *to* us. In reality you are constantly choosing, certainly within limits but still choosing. Your choices regarding psychosocial health habits are important; as much as possible you must make them consciously. We do not, of course, mean to imply that you are solely responsible for making changes even when you see what must be done. All of us need help, especially when the habits are deeply ingrained.

It is also important to remember that when we talk about psychosocial health habits affecting headaches we are not implying necessarily that your habits are not as healthy as your neighbor's or that they are in themselves psychological problems. Always remember that severe chronic headache is a physical illness that is affected by psychosocial factors rather than being ultimately caused by them. Therefore, we do not presume to tell you what you must change in your life. Rather, we ask you to engage in the process of becoming aware of what choices you are making with regard to psychosocial health habits and to honestly appraise how these choices seem to be interacting with your headaches. It may require you to do some experimenting with changes in the context of a comprehensive or multimodal treatment plan. Certainly you must do some careful observation. Haphazard self-reflection will disclose very little of psychosocial health habits that have become so ingrained as to be second nature.

The following are some common problem areas that you might do well to assess in your own life.

Inadequate Social Support

Social support is the availability of other people whom you want to associate with. It usually includes their ability and willingness to listen to your story—the story of your day, the story of your life, or anything in between. A mutual relationship is one in which you are asked, able, and willing to do the same for them. When such people aren't accessible, you can wind up feeling isolated and misunderstood, feelings that over time can contribute to internal tension and thus to headache. Relationships come in all levels of intimacy and have something to offer at each level. Building relationships takes place over time and requires working through the inevitable conflicts and disappointments.

Low Self-Esteem

This is a pervasive problem in our culture. Many people feel inadequate to the tasks in front of them, leading to a type of chronic anxiety. Others are ashamed of what they have done, what has happened to them, or what they have been able to achieve, creating a chronic sense of shame, disillusionment, or disappointment. Most of us carry these burdens inside, fearful of further humiliation if they become known. It is easy to see how the resulting anxiety or unhappiness could increase the risk of headaches. In addition, this way of thinking about yourself leads to skepticism that there is much you can do to take control of your headaches. Why should it be different from any other area of life? Fortunately, the techniques of sophisticated biobehavioral therapy can deal with broad issues like this as well as with the more concrete physical health habits and particular stress reactions. The choice to use it, discussed in Chapter 5, is yours.

Lack of Purpose in Life

Meaning in life—believing that you have something to accomplish and a reason for accomplishing it—is very important. Meaning may come from many sources. A common source is religious faith or a well-considered philosophy of life that places the apparently petty acts of day-to-day life in a larger framework. In this framework the days when nothing seems to work or on which there is great pain are more easily tolerated and understood. They bring wisdom rather than despair. You may still seem small in the grand scheme of things, but you are part of it all. With those of like mind, you are also part of a social group whose members support one another. Thus self-esteem and social support are enhanced.

An Unbalanced Life

Finally, imbalance among the many dimensions of your life can contribute to internal tension and other psychological distress, leading to greater headache risk. The most common source of imbalance in our lives is work versus play. This is not just a simple matter of how many hours you spend at the office. Work itself can be a great source of meaning for you and others. Play can become an end in itself, leading to a compulsive search for better toys or new thrills. Clues that suggest imbalance include becoming increasingly tense with spouse or children, feeling chained to the desk after everyone else has gone home, worrying about work not yet done, finding many things boring, or looking to new people to supply what has been missing in your life. You can achieve greater balance by setting limits based on choices about what you really want to do—this day, this week, this year.

In our patients we often see imbalance resulting from overemphasis on responsibilities—on the job or at home. If you have little sense of freedom and no hope that you can gain more freedom, you very well may feel stuck or trapped by the demands of others or of life. You may even feel guilty for chafing under your "lot." Always responding to the needs of others is a sure way to build resentment, depression, and anxiety. It may be very difficult to see the choices you have, and certainly it is equally important to see the limits on those choices, but professional assistance can be a great help in shaking up your tired and routine view of the world around you. You may find an opening to more joy in living and, in so doing, a respite from the burden of chronic headache.

In summary, we believe that reviewing psychosocial health habits is especially important and often overlooked in trying to manage chronic headache. However, we always consider them in the larger context of multimodal evaluation and treatment—recognizing that chronic headache is not ultimately *caused* by psychosocial factors or by any other class of triggering or contributing factors. We start with the realization that you have not chosen to be susceptible to chronic severe headache. It is an illness that in many cases seems to be inherited. It cannot even be controlled completely; there will always be times when headaches seem to come as they will, when chronic headache seems to have a "mind of its own." At the same time, you can work with your headache problem, taking responsibility to catch headaches early, respond effectively, identify triggers, modify them or your reactions to them, and work with general or contributing factors such as those outlined in this chapter. With help, you can do this, even if at first glance it seems too complex or too demanding. An ancient Chinese adage says that even a thousand-mile journey is begun with a single step. You must just start, with help, and the rest will follow as long as you persevere.

The model of care within which you will work must be broad enough to encompass all of what might be relevant to your headache and specific enough to use each of the particular treatments you might need, rather than offering only general advice. We will try to offer you that kind of model—the multimodal model of assessment and treatment—to help you begin assessing your own headache factors. To move yourself further along the road to control of your headaches, turn to Chapter 5.

✦

Identify Your Risk Factors: Some Preliminary Self-Help Techniques

Chapter 4 began with a discussion of factors difficult or impossible to control—family history, disease, hormonal changes—and continued toward ones it's more possible to control: medication use, muscle tension, internal tension, physical health habits, and psychosocial health habits. First you must learn which of these factors are most active in triggering or exacerbating your headache problem; then your treatment team can help you learn about and even develop ways to eliminate, minimize, or reduce the impact of the more controllable ones. This chapter shows how you can begin to identify your major risk factors on your own and take some self-help measures to eliminate them. Understanding the role you will play and taking some independent steps right away will only enhance your ability to collaborate with your treatment team.

Reducing the presence and impact of trigger factors will help you cut down on the number of headaches you have, and reversing negative contributing factors will make you a less congenial host to the headache syndrome by moving you toward a healthier lifestyle in general, one that maximizes vigor and enjoyment. Our experience suggests that when you feel more in control of your headaches you reap additional benefits as well. You'll probably find that you worry less about your health, feel more able to tackle life's challenges and more optimistic about the outcome. Simplified medication regimen, less muscle tension, greater sense of peace, better diet, more regular exercise, restful sleep, and more supportive social interaction—it can't hurt!

ASSESSING YOUR RISK OF HEADACHE: THE IMPORTANCE OF KEEPING RECORDS

Identifying the factors that may be affecting your risk of headache is one of the first and most important ways you can collaborate with your doctors and therapists to get your headaches under control. As you know from Chapter 1, this information is essential to developing an effective treatment plan. We believe that keeping a written record of some kind is the best way to approach this task. There are many potential factors affecting your headaches, and they interact with each other over time. Although critically important when they occur, there are few factors so powerful that they alone are sufficient to trigger a headache and that do so whenever they are present. Factors affecting headaches may act immediately, but they may also have delayed effects, making them harder to identify. You may not notice a headache right away, increasing the number of events that might have been responsible for its onset. In short, there are only a few factors that are obvious triggers of headache, ones easy to identify and eliminate. The real challenge, then, is to discover the more subtle offenders. Looking for these factors requires a systematic search over time. Keeping records is an essential part of this method.

In the comprehensive headache clinic the biobehavioral therapist is often an important participant in this search. The therapist encourages you to keep up the process of recordkeeping, helps you adapt the diary system to fit your particular style, reviews common triggers so you have an idea of what to look for, and scans the sheets each week, helping you look for likely suspects. In the diary you will be asked to keep track of not only when you have a headache but also how long the pain lasts and how quickly the pain moves from low to high intensity and back down. You will track activities that are commonly related to headache risk, like diet, mood, and the stress of the day. As you identify factors that seem particularly important in your unique headache syndrome, you will follow them with particular interest. Through this process, patterns will start to emerge. You will begin to see the relationships between factors and the onset or exacerbation of headache pain. Gradually you will become better able to determine how factors work together to increase the risk of headache. As you begin to identify the combinations of factors that contribute to your headaches, you will also see how they might be modified and how modifying one might actually make another, which you may not be able to change, less powerful.

If you can begin now to chart your headaches, you will be better able to help your physician or treatment team help you take control of your headaches. For one thing, you will be much better able to give your doctor an accurate picture of the current pattern of your headaches. In addition, you will be better able to describe accurately your current lifestyle and to offer useful ideas about which aspects of your lifestyle might be functioning as headache triggers. As one famous baseball wag put it, you will be surprised what you can see if you look.

In this chapter we offer a risk factors checklist you can use to help you focus on important information as you begin your recordkeeping. Although we use a standard form in our own clinic for maintaining the records, all clinics do it a little differently, and you also should modify the standard form to fit your particular preferences. What is most important is that you keep some kind of record and do it systematically rather than haphazardly. Later in the chapter you'll find other information that will give you more clues as to which factors may be pertinent to you. Appendix I gives additional checklists that can help you in your recordkeeping effort. The checklist on pages 63–65 is a set of questions you can address in keeping a daily diary of headache. (We suggest you enlarge this form when you photocopy it so that you will have more space to write in.)

The other side of recording risk factors is that you become a better observer of the headaches themselves. As you keep records and learn the rudiments of deep relaxation, you begin to notice headaches at lower levels of intensity, sometimes sensing muscle stiffness or other discomfort even before headache pain arises. Catching a headache early, of course, makes it easier for you to spot the factors that actually triggered it. When you're able to spot the very early signs of a headache, you have fewer events to sort through as possible triggers than you would have after more time had passed. Think about the investigator who comes on the crime scene minutes after the crime has been committed compared with the one who arrives several hours later; for the latter, the amount of extraneous "evidence" is very distracting. Catching a headache early will also serve you well in the course of treatment; the sooner you feel a headache coming on, the more quickly you can initiate treatment. Severe headache caught in its early stages is much easier to manage than when it has become very painful. If you see a truck rumbling toward you from two blocks away, you have many options; if you see the same truck two feet from you, there is little left to do.

RECORDING FACTORS IN HEADACHE

Date: _____

1. Check the "Today?" column for each factor you were aware of.
2. In the next column, note how this factor may have changed since yesterday.
3. In the last column, note how you plan to reduce this factor tomorrow.

	1. Today?	2. Change from yesterday?	3. How will I reduce tomorrow?
Use of any medication you haven't told your doctor about.			
Use of medication in excess of prescribed dose.			
Use of analgesics in excess of doctor's advice.			
Poor posture—e.g., forward neck, rounded shoulders, overly straight-up, rigid, tense, or braced			
Strain or overuse of muscle			
Bracing against pain			
Habitual frowning or raising eyebrows			
Grinding or clenching of teeth, habit of teeth touching			
Keeping shoulders up			
Limited or decreased range of motion in neck, shoulder, or upper-back area			
Imbalance in gait or sitting position			
Imbalance between muscle groups or pairs— side to side, front to back			
Trouble "letting go" of: anger			
anxiety			
frustration			

(cont.)

	1. Today?	2. Change from yesterday?	3. How will I reduce tomorrow?
Trouble "letting go" of: rage			
exhilaration			
depression			
guilt			
fear			
Too much worrying about things you can't affect			
Denying that problems exist			
Holding your breath			
Hyperventilating			
Shallow, rapid breathing			
Speaking too rapidly			
Lack of exercise			
Overly strenuous exercise			
Holding breath or muscle tension during exercise			
Too little sleep			
Too much sleep			
Trouble going to sleep or waking up			
Poor sleeping position— e.g., on the side, with too big a pillow			
Other interruptions of sleep cycle—apnea, nightmares			
Skipping meals			
Taking in too much fat, sugar, salt, caffeine, or alcohol			
Not drinking enough water			

(cont.)

	1. Today?	2. Change from yesterday?	3. How will I reduce tomorrow?
Taking in tyramine or MSG			
Too much dust or mold in house or workplace			
Overexposure to smoke or fumes			
Lighting that causes squinting			
Seating or work surfaces that lead to poor posture			
Lack of contact with family, friends, or co-workers			
Loneliness, dread, or boredom			
Thinking of self as victim or martyr			
Refusal to set specific goals			
Downgrading own character or abilities			
Procrastination			
Overperfectionism			
Taking on too much responsibility			
Feeling pressured			
Getting too busy to have time for self			
Not taking advantage of opportunities to develop interests and participate in activities within own capabilities and means			
Being too sensitive			
Being too aggressive or too passive			
Feeling uncomfortable with social skills			
Unspoken conflict or resentment			

Be persistent with your diary. Don't be discouraged if you have already kept a diary and found little benefit in it. Get help in designing your diary and reviewing it. One reason a treatment team is so valuable is that you have many pairs of experienced eyes to supplement your own. With their instruction and encouragement, your own powers of observation will be honed. At first, if you are new to the wild, you can tell very little about nearby animal life by looking at a given spot of land. When you stay there for a time with an experienced guide, you find yourself more able to read the clues to tell which animals have been by and how long ago. It is the same way with tracking your headache.

SELF-HELP IN IDENTIFYING RISK FACTORS

Here is what you can do to gather clues about your own risk factors and some steps you can take to begin eliminating them. Don't neglect any area, despite how unlikely it may seem to you.

Predisposition to Headache

Being aware of your family history of headache can give you a head start toward developing a plan to take control of your headache. If possible, ask your relatives about their headaches or what they know about the headaches of relatives who may be deceased. If an unusual type of headache runs in your family, the evaluation team may find this information very helpful. You also may be able to learn about factors influencing your headaches by investigating your family history. For example, if your parent or grandparent had a unique trigger, responded unusually to a certain medication, or benefited from a specific treatment, similar responses may be found in you. In the same way, use your experience to help you recognize headache patterns in your children if any of them have headaches.

On the other hand, remember that each person is unique. Don't force matters; it may be that your headache pattern will turn out to be completely different from that of your parents or children. Don't allow yourself to adopt a self-fulfilling prophecy of doom. If you have seen a family member suffer with headache, not receiving or seeking appropriate treatment, don't accept this fate for yourself. You can't change your family history or any predisposition to headache with which you may have been born, but you can change what you do about your headaches in the present. That's what taking control is all about.

The Menstrual Cycle

You can't avoid the hormonal changes associated with your menstrual cycle, it's true. But if you regularly have a headache with menstrual flow, you can use the predictability of this trigger to help you anticipate and reduce pain by responding before it ever shows its first signs.

With your diary, you can determine more precisely at what point in your menstrual cycle a headache is most likely to appear. If your menstrual cycle is reasonably regular, and if the headache occurs at the same point almost every month, days before headache begins you can begin reducing risk factors. You can use the suggestions in Appendix II to maximize your resistance to headaches, reducing physical and psychological stressors that might otherwise make you more vulnerable at this high-risk time.

In addition, you can work with your physician to use medications prior to the anticipated headache to reduce or even eliminate the pain. Usually, selected nonsteroidal anti-inflammatory medications will be used to prevent this type of headache. Finally, if all else fails, you still can use abortive medications promptly to cut off a severe headache. You are far from powerless with headaches triggered by hormonal changes associated with menstruation!

Medication

Medication plays an important role in the management of chronic headache. It would be difficult to imagine a comprehensive treatment plan in which some types of medication were not included. As important as it is, though, medication can also become part of the problem, especially for certain types of painkilling (analgesic) and abortive medications. This may seem strange to you; you may find it difficult to imagine that the same analgesics that have alleviated your suffering so often could actually be exacerbating it. It is the ultimate irony, but it is also a trap into which many headache sufferers have fallen. You'll learn more about so-called rebound headache in Chapter 6, but for now you can ask yourself a few preliminary questions to determine whether it's a potential factor in your case:

+ Does it seem as if your headaches are lasting longer?
+ Is it starting to seem that hardly a day goes by without some kind of headache?

+ Does it seem that you are waking with a headache more and more often?
+ Do you find yourself using some type of pain medication almost every day?
+ Have others worried about how much pain medication you are using?
+ Do you sometimes feel almost hooked on your medicine?
+ Do you find your pain increasing again just before you are scheduled for another dose of analgesic medication?
+ Do you find yourself using over-the-counter painkillers in addition to those prescribed by your doctor?
+ Has your use of analgesic medication increased gradually over a long period of time?
+ Do medications seem to work for a while and then wear off?

Again, your use of a diary is important. Many people are surprised to see just how much of various medications they are using once they begin to record it systematically. Turning to medication is very natural. The headache is painful; you reach for what you can to help reduce the pain. The trap is so subtle because most headache patients are not "drug seekers," but they can become desperate for relief. Desperation can lead anyone to do even what he or she knows is not ultimately healthy. Look at this area honestly and stay aware of how, when, and why you are using medicines.

Muscle Tension

As you now know, muscle irritation is very common among those with chronic headache, and most often it is found in the muscles of the upper body—shoulders, neck, and face. These muscles may have become irritated from chronic tension, from some injury, or even from bracing against the pain of the headache itself. However, many people do not realize their muscles are painfully irritated until they undergo medical examination. The physician or physical therapist may press against the muscles, causing you to flinch. You may believe at first that this occurs only because the doctor or therapist put so much pressure on the muscle, but usually it is your muscles that are "talking back." This kind of soreness with normal pressure is one indication that the muscles are irritated. There are other indications as well. Do you experience chronic stiffness or aching in the muscles of your upper body? Do you feel muscle pain even after prolonged postures of one type or another? Do you feel pain with large movements of your jaw or neck? Are you aware of any knots or tender points in your muscles? Can you move your neck or jaw less than you once could? If you can answer yes to some of these questions, muscle tension may be a risk factor for you as it is for so many chronic headache patients. However it occurred, it may now be a factor that is triggering or exacerbating headache.

To zero in on its exact location and effect, however, you'll need the help of your treatment team. During the initial evaluation at a comprehensive headache center, you would be asked about symptoms such as those just mentioned. Doctors will press the muscles of your upper body to see whether you have pain from normal pressure. You will be asked to move your neck and jaw to see if you have full range of movement and if you can make the movements without causing pain. Sometimes, in the course of this type of evaluation or afterward, you will actually notice that a headache has been triggered. Although this is unfortunate, and the headache should be treated promptly, it is also important information indicating that muscle irritation is indeed actively working to keep your headache syndrome going. Treating chronically sore muscles can be tricky, but it is a critical part of the comprehensive treatment plan.

Health Habits

We suggested in Chapter 4 that health habits like exercise, sleep, physical environment, and diet are often factors in headaches. In some cases they may be triggering headaches; however, in this context we are concerned especially with their role as contributing or contextual factors, making you generally more vulnerable to the headache syndrome.

Here's where your own efforts can really make a difference. Only you can observe your personal habits intimately enough to uncover all possible factors. Compare your observations of self-care in these areas against the ideals suggested by your treatment team and begin experimenting with changes. Do this as part of a comprehensive treatment plan, but a little at a time, and you won't feel overwhelmed by the task. Make changes in the ideal plan to suit your particular style, and you may actually stick with it over the long haul!

Is it worth the trouble? We have plenty of evidence that it is. Sometimes identifying and then modifying an important health habit affecting headaches proves to be the key to taking control, working in tandem with other parts of the treatment plan. For example, in one study adding attention to dietary factors affecting headaches remarkably increased the effect of a treatment plan that previously included only stress reduction and biofeedback techniques. As always, we believe that this willingness to combine many approaches to headache management at the same time is the key to successful control of chronic headache syndromes.

Use the following questions to help you determine which health habits and environmental factors may be worth a closer look in your headache problem. *Yes* answers indicate a factor that might be playing a role in triggering, exacerbating, or maintaining your headaches.

- Do I use tobacco?
- Do I exercise less than three times a week?
- Do I often feel physically sluggish?
- Am I so tired when I get home from work that I just can't do anything but slump in a soft chair?
- Do I have pain when I do certain types of exercise?
- Do I go to sleep at a different time each night?
- Do I have trouble getting to sleep?
- Does my sleep seem interrupted or of poor quality?
- Is my sleeping position uncomfortable, or is it one that is not recommended for individuals with head or neck pain (sleeping on my stomach or with too big a pillow)?
- Do I wake at a different time each morning?
- Do I get up much later on some mornings?
- Do I wake up before I want to many mornings?
- Do I have trouble waking up?
- Am I sleepy often during the daytime?
- Do I skip meals?
- Do I overeat to the point of feeling stuffed and sluggish?
- Have I noticed weight gain?
- How far over my target weight am I?
- Is my appetite unpredictable?
- Is my diet high in fat, salt, and sugar?
- Do I drink less than six to eight glasses of water a day?
- Do I average more than two alcoholic drinks a day?
- Do I drink alcoholic beverages every day to help me relax?
- Do I typically drink several caffeinated beverages (coffee, tea, soda) a day?
- If I don't have these beverages, do I feel achy, tired, irritable, or have a headache?

- ✦ Do I use over-the-counter medications for headache (or other reasons) that contain caffeine, more than two to three days a week?
- ✦ Do I have a headache when I don't use these medicines?
- ✦ Do I regularly notice symptoms of allergic reactions (like congestion, sneezing, runny nose, tearing eyes, bloodshot eyes) in environments where I spend a lot of time?
- ✦ Do I have such reactions to certain odors to which I am often exposed, like tobacco, cleaning products, or strong perfumes?
- ✦ Do I experience eye strain in work or home environments, perhaps due to poor lighting conditions?
- ✦ In my work situation, at home or the office, are the chairs and work surfaces comfortable for me?
- ✦ Does my work position require that I maintain a single position for long periods of time?
- ✦ Do I experience strain in my upper back or neck muscles from leaning forward for long periods?
- ✦ Do I frequently hold a telephone between my ear and shoulder to free my hands?
- ✦ Does my work area seem unpleasantly crowded or noisy?
- ✦ Am I exposed directly to blasts of heated or cooled air from the climate-control system?

This list may seem long, but there are actually many more questions you could ask. These illustrate some of the areas that are often problematic in people with chronic severe headache. More important, they help you realize more fully the need to be sensitive to your headache pattern and the factors that affect it.

You may feel overwhelmed by the number of possible factors, or you may believe that you would not have time for anything else if you started observing in all these areas. Actually the scheme is not as impractical as it may seem, and you are not going to become obsessed with your health. The key is making observation a habit and self-regulation of headache (and of your health in general) a matter of course. At first you use the diary to shake you from your usual inattention, but after a time you find that you have learned a new level of awareness in the course of your daily life. It becomes second nature to notice changes in your body, identify factors that influenced the changes, and make adjustments. It is no more than learning to live harmoniously in body, mind, and spirit.

Once you have identified problem areas, taking action is the next step. For some factors avoiding or eliminating the habit is the key. Naturally, accomplishing this may be more difficult than talking about it. Caffeine overuse, whether in beverages or medications, may require tapering to avoid a period of painful headache. Smoking really serves no useful purpose but is a devilishly hard habit to break.

In other areas you may need to develop new habits that are more consistent with headache management and general good health. Developing a new habit is not impossible, but it does require persistence. Consider exercise, for example. If you are relatively sedentary—like the legendary couch potato—it will be important to set aside time for an appointment with yourself to exercise. Get your doctor's approval for the regimen you select, then find ways to make it easy for you to do. Consider what will work for you. Is it having a machine in the house or inviting an exercise partner to help get you out of your chair at the appointed time? If exercise causes pain, select a new form that will not jar your head and neck and will not increase the load on your heart and blood vessels so severely. You may find that *gentle* aerobic exercise can actually reduce minor headache pain.

Sleep takes up about one-third of our lives, and an important one-third it is. Start by making sure that you have regular times to go to bed and to wake, varying by no more than an hour or two even on weekends. If you have a problem getting to sleep or waking too early, be sure that you consult your treatment team for specific behavioral or medication treatment; it is available. If you work different shifts, consider consulting a sleep expert for the best ways to compensate. Finally, get enough sleep. So many people seem to worry that they will waste time by sleeping or feel too pressured by their schedules to allow enough time in bed. If you recognize yourself here, take a hard look. The quality of your waking life may hang in the balance.

Diet

This health habit is worth special consideration because, as we've mentioned, healthy eating habits are important to reducing your general vulnerability to headaches. Among other things we've encouraged you to eat regularly scheduled meals, eat more vegetables than meats, reduce salt, and avoid overeating.

In addition to the overall role of healthy dietary habits, food can be a potent trigger of headaches. (When we say *food* here, we include

beverages and additives.) The subject is complicated and has been difficult to study scientifically. Most headache professionals recognize the
important role that diet plays in headache syndromes, but the nature of
that role and the way to approach it in treatment are the subject of some
controversy.

It is certainly fair to state that many patients are definitely affected
by at least some foods. Tyramine is a substance found in many foods,
including aged cheeses and meats, and many forms of alcoholic beverages, to which many headache persons react adversely. Monosodium
glutamate, a food additive more commonly known as MSG, is also
frequently reported as a headache trigger. Not all headache patients,
however, report food triggers, and those patients who do seem sensitive
to food do not all respond to the same foods. Even those who definitely
seem to identify food triggers may not always respond to that food with
a headache. One reason may be that the level of tyramine or other
offending substances can vary widely in different selections of the same
food. Also, under varying conditions the same food may have different
effects. For example, eating a food known to trigger headaches many
hours after your last meal—on an empty stomach—seems to be riskier
than eating that food in the course of a meal.

Nevertheless, there are some practical steps you can take to identify
foods that may be headache triggers for you.

Food Diary

The food diary can be part of the overall headache diary or a project
of its own. To keep a food diary, simply write down whatever you have
to eat or drink and the approximate time of day. As you review your
entries over any given day, check for foods that are known to trigger
headaches in many people. Table 2 presents a brief list of foods that
we find frequently related to headaches among our patients. There is
also a more extensive list under "Elimination Diet." Note whether a
headache often follows your eating such foods, usually within several
hours. If you have trouble tracking down a cause for your headaches,
but you do find some of these trigger foods in your regular diet,
consider eliminating them for the time being, until your headaches are
under better control. Then you can reintroduce them one at a time,
starting with those that you think are least likely to trigger headaches.
Proceed gradually so that you will note if you have a reaction to a
particular food. If you think you do but are not sure, try it again; it is

TABLE 2. Foods Commonly Associated with Headaches

Food additives

* MSG (monosodium glutamate)
  Yellow cheddar cheese (colored with annatto)
  Nitrates and nitrites (found in processed meats like ham

Tyramine-containing foods (partial list)

* Red wines and most other alcoholic beverages
* Aged cheeses and meats
  Nuts
  Milk products
  Other foods
  Chocolate
* Caffeine (usually during withdrawal)

Occasional reports

  Aspartame (NutraSweet)
  Eggs
  Chicken livers
  Canned figs
  Onion
  Shellfish
  Pickled herring
  Pods of broad beans

* = Most common triggers.

hard to draw a conclusion from a single incident since other factors may have affected your reaction.

When you keep a food diary as part of an overall headache diary, you can also work backward from headaches. Whenever you have recorded the onset of a significant headache, review the record for all the foods taken in over the previous twenty-four hours. Check especially for the foods known to trigger headaches, but keep an open mind; you may have an unusual reaction. If you find that a particular food is frequently present in your diet before a headache, especially if that food is otherwise known as a trigger of headaches, consider eliminating that food as suggested. This process takes time and can be frustrating; however, your biobehavioral therapist, dietician, or nurse will often be very helpful to you in systematically tracking down food–headache relationships.

Use Table 2 along with your food diary or comprehensive headache diary.

Elimination Diet

A more comprehensive approach to identifying food triggers is to eliminate all possible offending foods from your diet, substituting with comparable foods not likely to cause headaches. This is much more disruptive of your lifestyle, and many of the foods eliminated will turn out to have little to do with your particular headache problem. However, the tests that purport to determine "food allergies" do not seem to be much more specific or any more reliable at picking out food triggers of headaches.

If you eliminate many different foods from your meals, you must be careful to maintain a well-balanced diet with adequate nutrients. A dietician can provide important support in making such a radical change to your diet, which should be done under the general supervision of your physician.

You may use Table 3 to adjust your diet. Avoid all foods in the "Foods to avoid" column, substituting foods from the "Foods to try" column. Once you have gotten used to this diet, reintroduce "Foods to avoid" items that you especially like, one at a time. Use each food for a few days and see if it seems to trigger a headache. If it does, you may have identified a food that is powerful enough to trigger a headache under most conditions. You should continue to avoid it. If it doesn't, you have discovered a food you may be able to eat, but continue to observe it to ensure that it is not a more subtle offender.

In summary, following the advice of health professionals in our everyday health habits is always a good idea—but perhaps especially for headache sufferers. The choices we routinely make in exercise, sleep, diet, and environment make a difference. Good health habits alone may not relieve headaches, but poor ones are highly likely to result in more frequent headaches.

Internal Tension and Psychosocial Habits

Along with muscle tension, internal tension (arousal) might be considered one of the final common pathways of headaches. No matter what triggers a particular headache attack or what type of headache is triggered, muscle tension and/or internal tension are often experienced or observed before headache pain begins. They are very often part of the series of events that culminates in a headache. For that reason almost anyone who has headaches can benefit from increased

TABLE 3. Food Substitutions

Foods to avoid	Foods to try
Beverages	
Most alcoholic beverages, especially red wine, beer	Water, fruit juices
Coffee or tea	Decaffeinated coffee or teas
Coke, Pepsi, other colas, Mountain Dew, Mello Yello	7-UP, Sprite, ginger ale, carbonated water, root beer, decaffeinated colas
Cocoa or other chocolate drinks	Postum and other grain drinks
Dairy products	
Whole milk, buttermilk, cream, sour cream	Skim or 1 percent milk, yogurt, frozen yogurt, sherbet
Aged cheeses in general, cheddar, mozzarella, Camembert, Tilsiter, Roquefort, Gouda, Harzer cheese, Emmenthal	Other soft cheeses, cottage cheese
Meats	
Beef liver, hot dogs, salami, ham, bacon, lunch meats, summer sausages, other cured or processed meats, canned meats or meat pies	Fresh or frozen meat
Poultry	
Chicken liver	Fresh or frozen poultry
Fish	
Pickled herring, shellfish, dried smoked fish, mackerel, anchovy, sardine, tunny	Fresh or frozen fish not otherwise listed, canned salmon, tuna
Vegetables	
Most beans	String (green) beans
Onions, peas, olives, pickles, sauerkraut, spinach, tomatoes	Asparagus, beets, carrots, squash, corn, zucchini, broccoli, lettuce, potatoes
Grains	
Sourdough bread	Whole-wheat and rye breads, rice, pasta, English muffins, melba toast, bagels, matzoh, most cereals
Soups	
Soups containing MSG or yeast, soups made with bouillon cubes	Homemade soups (reading labels of canned soups may not always help— MSG can be present without being clearly stated)

(cont.)

TABLE 3 *(cont.)*

Foods to avoid	Foods to try
	Fruits
Citrus fruits, bananas, figs, raisins, papaya, kiwi fruit, plums, pineapple, avocado, red grapes, raspberries	Prunes, apples, cherries, white grapes, apricots, peaches, pears
	Desserts and snacks
Chocolates, licorice, nuts, seeds	Hard candy, cakes, cookies, Jell-O
Peanut butter	Jam, jelly, honey
	Additives and condiments
MSG, soy sauce, marinades, extra salt, yeast products, aspartame (NutraSweet)	White vinegar, salad dressing

awareness of muscle and internal tension and from effective techniques to relax them.

It has become increasingly obvious in the scientific research that using techniques to reduce stress succeeds in reducing the number of headaches for many people over long periods of time; it allows medication use to be reduced as well. So, if becoming sensitive to internal tension, learning to relax, and reducing stress in everyday life seem like formidable tasks, keep in mind that the rewards can be substantial. Although self-help techniques are clearly valuable and often effective, professional help can be very important in this effort. Working with a professional lends support, encouragement, motivation, and a practiced pair of eyes to identify the sources of stress you might otherwise miss. People often do not recognize the sources of stress that are most prevalent in their lives simply because they become accustomed to them. Certain individuals are almost constantly tense but do not think of themselves that way simply because tension is ever present and thus unremarkable. Biofeedback techniques can help you become more sensitive to the physical changes associated with internal and muscle tension and tell you when the relaxation is indeed producing physical changes, not just an illusion of relaxation. Behavioral simulation of stressful situations allows you to practice just shy of the real thing.

Among the factors leading to muscle tension and internal tension are the psychosocial habits. Your psychosocial health habits are really a series of choices you are making in everyday life, but they may be so ingrained that you hardly think of them as options. "It's just the way I am" and "That's just the way things are" are common perceptions that keep us going in the same old ruts. Your treatment team will help you examine the choices you are making if you are willing to take a fresh look at your life and your relationships. In this way you may be able to correct repetitive problems that lead to tension rather than working only with the aftereffects, in the form of muscle tension or internal tension.

Let's review a few of the areas in which people very often have dysfunctional psychosocial health habits. Consider social support. Do you do so much for others, but no one seems willing to do for you? Does it seem that you must do all the bending while others get their way? Are you always asking others to go out but never seem to be asked yourself? Of course the others in your life also play a role in the choices they make; you are not responsible for everything that happens. Very often, though, you are acting in ways that encourage the very patterns you hate so much. This is not a blaming statement—quite the opposite in fact. It is a freeing statement. If you are responsible for some of what you hate, the good news is that you also have the power to make it different. Perhaps you need new skills, like assertiveness, or reduction in anxiety with other people. There are many effective therapies to help you make the necessary changes.

Similarly, low self-esteem leads you to negative thoughts about your inherent value or the success of your efforts. In our age, many people go through life with a vague sense of anxiety, feeling "not good enough." You may expect that others will not be interested in you, and that expectation may actually make it more difficult for you to make a good impression on others. By holding back because you expect failure or rejection you can find yourself in a vicious circle of disappointment and further negative expectations. You are left only with the cold comfort of knowing that your hypothesis was correct. Raising self-esteem is not simply a matter of willpower. You need feedback from others to see that the world is not necessarily as you see it now and encouragement to try out other possible ways of being and doing. Your first step is to take the chance with professionals and friends to talk about the experience and consider the alternatives.

Many individuals lose, for a short time or for much of their adult lives, a sense of purpose or meaning in life. There can be many reasons for losing this sense of meaning, and sometimes it is an important stage of development, coming to see your life and relationships in an entirely new light. However, chronic lack of meaning is a draining condition, sapping energy and will. Life seems to drag on without purpose. If you lack this sense of purpose or meaning, it is important to consider the choices that you have made and are continuing to make every day. You may have the *feeling* of no control over your reality, but the fact is that your behavior and your thinking pattern are at each moment either moving you farther along the path to meaninglessness or moving you back to identifying the context in which your life plays a role in the world.

Finally, balance in our lives, usually between "play" and work, can be hard to maintain. The right balance is a personal matter. Some of us can work long hours but find ourselves refreshed rather than drained by the effort. Learning to pace yourself while working is one factor, and developing the sense of appropriate and realistic control over your work is another. Are you a "people person" who thrives in the company of others, most comfortable in a family group or with friends? Or do you need more time to yourself to calm and recharge yourself? What is important is that you take the time to listen to your body and your mind, to hear if you are stressed, and to consider what needs to change. Listening to the feedback of family and friends is also important; balance is not just a condition to be achieved inside; the solution must include your social unit. If you are bored by inactivity, is the answer to keep busy, or are there things inside or in your relationships from which you are running? If you are a high achiever, are you simply expressing your creativity, or are you only avoiding failure? These are the kinds of questions that you must pose to yourself and that your biobehavioral therapist, family, and friends can help you answer.

Don't be afraid to explore this portion of the path toward headache control. Although most comprehensive headache clinics consider the psychological professionals very important members of the team, sometimes headache sufferers are defensive about the psychosocial parts of their evaluation and treatment. They may have encountered a doctor who told them that the headache was "all in their head" or that they were a "psych case." They may believe, without really saying so, that if there are psychological problems then the headache is not real or is not a serious medical problem. If you have these concerns, the answer is not to avoid or play down the psychological part of treatment but to confront your distorted beliefs. Of course, chronic headache is a medical problem. It is in effect a chronic illness that must be treated. Medicine plays an important role in any treatment plan. Physical therapy is often important. Other medical specialists may have a role to play. However, there is no denying the fact that headaches are also very often triggered by psychosocial stress.

There is no fairness about it, but the fact that you are predisposed to headaches may mean that you can't get away with even the normal amount of stress in your life. This is not necessarily only a curse. You might see it also as an invitation and an opportunity, a chance to recognize and take charge of areas in your life that, while not disabling, are keeping you from full expression of your potential. The good news is that relatively brief biobehavioral therapy often can help you overcome the dysfunctional psychosocial habits that may be increasing muscle tension and internal tension and thus adding to your headaches. It is another part of working with your treatment team to take control of your headaches.

✦   THE CASE OF KAREN L., PART 2

In Chapter 4 we introduced Karen L. and the main risk factors that were identified in her chronic headache syndrome. Karen's doctors made the obvious recommendations: she was asked to increase the hours of sleep she got each night, schedule gentle aerobic exercise three times a week, eat regularly, drink less cola and more water, and stop smoking. As her treatment continued, Karen's biobehavioral therapist would help her in these efforts, keeping records with her and developing behavioral strategies to assist in changing habits. We will describe those efforts in detail in the following chapters, which discuss the individual modalities of treatment available to chronic headache sufferers. This chapter should have helped you begin to review the factors that may influence your own headaches. If you elect to pursue treatment in a comprehensive headache clinic, we feel confident that your physician, psychologist, and therapists will be able to offer specific, individual help with whatever choices you face.

✦

CHAPTER 6

Use Medication Wisely

You may recall that when Karen L. came to our headache clinic for help with chronic daily headaches, she arrived armed with a fistful of medications. She had prescriptions for an analgesic compound containing aspirin, caffeine, and a barbiturate and for amitriptyline, a tricyclic antidepressant that can act as a preventive medication for chronic headache. On her own, Karen had begun using the analgesic medication more often than the prescription called for and was supplementing it with over-the-counter painkillers as often as several times per day. She also had a prescription for a medication to clear her congestion and an estrogen supplement since she had undergone a hysterectomy. Despite the medicine prescribed for her pain, her headaches were occurring almost daily; they were often severe, even debilitating.

Sadly, Karen's case is not unusual. Sometimes, despite the best intentions and efforts of both patient and physician, chronic headache persists. Sometimes the wealth of pharmacological resources available to manage headaches can actually, and paradoxically, make the problem worse. There are few things more discouraging to chronic headache patients than to find themselves in this trap fashioned of desperation, anxiety, and frustration. This chapter explains how to avoid the pitfall of excessive medication use and moves you farther along the road to controlling your headaches.

If you have already been discouraged by the failure of medication alone to control your frequent severe headaches, you'll be heartened to learn that there is hope for you—in other modalities of therapy and in wise selection and moderate use of medicine. If you find yourself resisting this information or skeptical of suggestions that less and more selective use of medication rather than a more drastic prescription might

tive use of medication rather than a more drastic prescription might actually be part of the blueprint for better control of headaches, we ask only that you read on with an open mind. With chronic severe headache there is just no future in using painkilling medications like so many hand grenades, tossing them down your throat in a desperate effort to knock out the enemy headache. The aim of this chapter is to show that effective use of medication in the management of headaches is a complex matter, requiring your full attention and participation. It takes time to allow some medications to work and to find the optimal combination of medicine and other therapies to manage your pain. Whatever your current orientation, this chapter very well may change your perspective.

TEN PRINCIPLES FOR WISE
USE OF MEDICATION

The first and overriding rule of thumb is to think of medication as *one* of the important therapies in managing your headache. Although it is a critical part of the overall plan, in the case of chronic headache medication cannot cure. When asked to do the whole job alone, medication-only treatment may not be as effective as you would like with very frequent headaches.

Medication is the first of four modes of headache therapy that we discuss in Chapters 6–9 of this book. Whether you have consulted only your primary care physician, been to see a headache specialist, or are seeking help from a comprehensive headache clinic, your physician may recommend various types of drugs known to be effective in breaking the vicious circle of biological factors that culminate in the painful attacks of migraine, cluster, or tension headaches. Used *wisely*, these medications are a potent force in controlling headache. Here are some principles to guide you in their wise and conservative use:

1. Know Yourself

This simple but basic principle applies here as it does in so many areas of our lives. With regard to control of your headaches, it is essential that you be aware of the underlying and usually unspoken beliefs that guide you in making treatment decisions. Your attitude toward medication is one of these underlying beliefs that is particularly important. Do you think of medication as the only real treatment? If your doctor does not give you a pill, do you feel you have not been treated? Do you expect medication to take care of the whole problem? Are you conservative about taking medicine, preferring to take it only when necessary and in minimal doses? Or are you more daring, willing to experiment and less cautious about what you take or about sticking to a particular regimen? As you know by now, we believe that (all other things being equal) the less medication you must take, the better for your body. In general, we've found that those with a conservative attitude toward medication, with reasonable expectations of what it can (and can't) do, are more open at the start to trying multimodal therapy. Before you read on, ask yourself where you stand.

2. Stay Focused on the Collaborative Approach

If you are trapped in a self-defeating spiral, using more and more medicine but feeling more frequent and severe pain, you may feel discouraged and frustrated. Both you and your physician may feel helpless to do anything about the pain. At its extreme this situation leads to mutual blame: your physician may start to think of you as a drug seeker, while you may wonder if your physician cares or is competent.

It is actually quite easy to fall into the trap of medication overuse. Your physician wants most of all to help, and you want very much to control the pain. If medicine seems to be the only tool available, you will use it as much as you can. When it fails, however, blaming each other only increases the problem. The way out is to honestly confront reality. Intentions aside, you are not getting the results that you want. Medication use is increasing; your headaches are not under control. It is not reasonable for you to simply demand new or more medication to "fix" the problem. At that point you and your physician can begin to think creatively *together* about other solutions. This may mean stepping back for a fuller assessment of the problem, getting additional consultations, and/or seeking referral to a comprehensive headache clinic. You begin to consider your role in managing this chronic condition, taking the active approach rather than passively waiting to be cured.

3. Be Realistic

Wise use of medication also means recognizing what it can and can't do. Medication is not a cure for chronic headache. It is an important part of the treatment plan, but only one among several modes of control. In the case of frequent severe headache medication delivered in safe doses often cannot eliminate headache altogether and all at once. It will serve as part of the plan, helping to reduce severity, frequency, and duration of pain. Medication usually plays its part most effectively when it is not asked to carry the whole load, when you allow it to work alongside one or more of the other modes of therapy we discuss in Chapters 7–9—modes that offer other ways of recognizing and controlling the factors that may contribute to your headache.

Also, recognize that prescribing medication for headaches can be as much clinical art as science. While your physician knows which medications usually are effective for various types of headaches, medicines affect individual people differently. What is effective in reducing even very similar headaches for someone you know may not work for you. Side effects are difficult to predict. What one person can take with no problems another may react to with unacceptable discomfort. Often your physician can only tell you what problems to look out for after starting a particular medication and try to be responsive if you do have problems. It may turn out that a medication that is perfectly effective for many people will not control your headaches. In that case you may have to try a series of medicines systematically, giving each enough time to work, before you find the right one for you.

It's not unusual to have unrealistic expectations for medication. All of us wish, if we must be sick, for a sickness that can be readily diagnosed and cured. Unfortunately, chronic severe headache is not such a condition. It takes patience to avoid the frustration and fear that can lead to medication overuse. On the other hand, you have a right to expect your physician to explain clearly to you why he or she is trying a particular medicine, what it is expected to do, what side effects to watch for, and when it will be clear whether it is helping. Being willing to try several medicines does not mean allowing yourself to be led through an indefinite and unexplained series of trials. Prescribing may not be exact, but it can be systematic.

4. Stay Informed

Make sure you understand the terms your physician uses when discussing medication. Know, for instance, that an analgesic is a painkiller, while a prophylactic medicine has a preventive effect. An abortive medication stops the headache once it has already begun. When you don't understand a term your physician uses, don't hesitate to ask for an explanation. Let your physician or other members of the treatment team know if you need a simpler explanation or would benefit from written material.

In addition to asking your physician, you can seek out information on your own. Because you are reading this book, we already know that you take the time to find self-help books on headaches. There are also self-help books on medications themselves. Your pharmacist is an expert source of information on the interaction of medications with other medicines, foods, or diseases.

This chapter also provides an overview of the medications usually prescribed for the main types of headaches, including a summary in chart form (see Table 4, later). Use all these sources of information to boost your knowledge and ability to be an active partner in treatment, but remember that your physician is the authoritative source and final reference for any decisions regarding medication.

Another aspect of staying informed is making sure you bring up the questions that are important to you. You don't need to be a wallflower, nor do you have to question your physician in a challenging or angry way. An active and questioning patient is playing his or her role as a member of the treatment team. Whenever your doctor prescribes a new medication, be sure you know the answers to these questions:

- ✦ What is this medication supposed to do?
- ✦ What are the possible side effects?
- ✦ How soon after beginning to take the medication should I notice a change or an effect?
- ✦ Should I notice an effect with each dose, or is it a cumulative effect?
- ✦ Is this the kind of medicine I should take regularly or just when I have pain? If the latter, should I take it as soon as I notice pain or only when I know this will be a severe headache?
- ✦ What is the maximum amount I should take per day and per week? Is there a limit to the number of days per week I should use this medicine?
- ✦ Should I take this medicine with meals or on an empty stomach? Are there any other specific instructions for how to take the medicine?
- ✦ Are there any potential problems with taking this medication over the long term?
- ✦ Should any tests be done to monitor how much of the medicine

is getting to my bloodstream or to monitor possible damage to kidneys, liver, or other organs?

+ Will this medication conflict with other medications that I am taking, any foods or beverages I might consume, or any other medical condition?

+ How will this medication affect pregnancy [if you are a woman of childbearing age]?

+ How long will I need to take this medication?

+ Should the dose be altered for certain circumstances? (For example, if no headache occurs for several weeks, should I continue to take this medicine, or should I discontinue it and restart it another time?)

+ What is the cost?

+ Is there an equally effective generic medication?

5. Follow Instructions to the Letter

Once you know what to do with your medication, do it. This may seem like obvious advice, but it often goes unheeded. Medicine like an antidepressant that takes two or three weeks to have its maximum impact may be discontinued after a few days without benefit. Preventive medicine of this type is meant to be taken each day, regardless of headache activity, but sometimes we find people using it only when they have pain. With analgesic or abortive medication, when headache is not responding to treatment there is a great temptation to take more medicine than prescribed or to use it more days per week than the limit established. Some people add over-the-counter painkillers without consulting their physician in the belief that over-the-counter medication "doesn't count."

Some errors result from the fear and desperation that are associated with headaches that are not responding to treatment. These mistakes are understandable, but they are also detrimental to comprehensive headache management. We know that using more and more medication sometimes backfires, having the opposite effect of that intended: the headaches become worse. Analgesic-induced headache is discussed in full later in this chapter.

Other mistakes occur just from lack of understanding. With everything you have to think about when you visit your physician, it's common not to hear or remember all the instructions given. Therefore it's always wise to ask for medication instructions in writing. Similarly, ask your pharmacist for any handouts available on the drug, its effects and side effects. If there are discrepancies with what you understand to be your physician's instructions, call your doctor for clarification. Refer also to the other sources of information you have compiled on medicines for headaches. Knowing this type of information helps you work with your doctor to get the most from medication while avoiding potential problems.

6. Notice and Record the Effects of the Medication

The therapeutic effects of medications are difficult to predict for the individual. For that reason your observations of the effect of the medicine, for good or bad, are very important. To be a good observer, you must be systematic. Any good scientist learns first to distrust his or her casual observation. We can be influenced remarkably by what we expect to see. If you are convinced that a medicine will cause terrible side effects, you are much more likely to have them. If you think a medicine is going to cure you no matter what, it is much more likely to work at least in the short term. Use your diary (see Chapter 5) to record all the changes and effects you notice after taking a dose of the medicine and also over the longer term. Don't assume that your doctor knows any of the details just because the medication is supposed to work that way. Be precise and comprehensive. This method will help you avoid the pitfalls of inaccurate or incomplete observations and will help you get to the right medicine more quickly.

7. Know the Side Effects

Side effects are also difficult to predict. If you read only the official descriptions of a medication, you probably would never use another. These descriptions list all possible side effects, most of which occur in only a small minority of patients when the medication is used as recommended. On the other hand, they do highlight that such side effects, some of them serious, can occur. As we have mentioned, no potent medication, whether prescription or over-the-counter, is completely safe. That is why we continue to encourage you not to use more medication than is necessary and to use other therapies to reduce the need for medication. Your physician depends on you to understand what side effects your medicines might produce and which should be reported immediately. Ask if you don't receive full information on this subject.

Table 4 lists some of the side effects we have seen most often at our

TABLE 4. Selected Medications for Headache

Generic name	Selected trade names	Cautions and possible side effects[*]
I. Analgesics and nonsteroidal anti-inflammatory drugs		
Simple analgesics		
Aspirin	Bayer, Bufferin, Ecotrin, house brands	Avoid with ulcer; may irritate stomach
Acetaminophen	Tylenol, Datril, Anacin-3, house brands	High doses may lead to liver/kidney problems
Analgesics with caffeine		
Aspirin compounds	Anacin, Excedrin	Same as aspirin; with frequent use, caffeine may increase risk of rebound headache
Nonsteroidal anti-inflammatory drugs		
Ibuprofen	Motrin, Advil, Nuprin, house brands	Avoid with ulcer; may irritate stomach, lead to dizziness; indomethacin may cause headache
Indomethacin	Indocin	
Naproxen	Naprosyn, Anaprox, Aleve	
Analgesics with caffeine and barbiturate		
Aspirin compounds	Fiorinal, generic	With frequent use, barbiturate and caffeine increase risk of rebound headache; also nausea, drowsiness, dizziness
Acetaminophen compounds	Fioricet, Esgic, Medigesic	
Analgesics with narcotic		
Aspirin compounds with codeine	Fiorinal	Risk of addiction from narcotics, nausea, vomiting, drowsiness, constipation
with oxycodone	Percodan	Light-headedness, dizziness, sedation, nausea, risk of abuse
with propoxyphene	Darvon-N	
Acetaminophen compounds with oxycodone	Percocet, Tylox	
Narcotics		
Butorphanol	Stadol (nasal spray)	Risk of addiction, nausea

(cont.)

TABLE 4 *(cont.)*

Generic name	Selected trade names	Cautions and possible side effects[*]
Narcotics (cont.)		
Meperidine	Demerol	Avoid with MAO inhibitor; risk of addiction, dizziness, nausea, sedation, decrease in breathing rate and volume, increased sweating; may be given by injection
Morphine		Risk of addiction, dizziness, nausea, sedation; usually given by injection

II. Abortive medications		
Ergot derivatives		
Ergotamine	Ergostat, Medihaler Ergotamine Aerosol	Avoid with heart, vascular, liver, or kidney disease, or high blood pressure
Ergotamine with caffeine	Cafergot, Wigraine	Same as ergotamine; caffeine may be headache factor; overuse may cause poor circulation in fingers and toes
Ergotamine with barbiturate	Bellergal-S	Same as ergotamine; also drowsiness
Dihydroergotamine	DHE-45	Same as ergotamine
Steroids		
Prednisone	Deltasone	May lead to nausea, ulcers, weakness, lowered resistance to infection, high blood pressure, avoid with any infection
Dexamethasone	Decadron	Same as prednisone
Others		
Sumatriptan	Imitrex	Avoid with heart disease, high blood pressure, may lead to pain at injection site

(cont.)

TABLE 4 *(cont.)*

Generic name	Selected trade names	Cautions and possible side effects*
Others (cont.)		
Acetaminophen, isometheptene, dichloralphenazone	Midrin, Isocom	Avoid with MAO inhibitor, glaucoma, or heart, liver, or kidney disease; may lead to dizziness
Prochlorperazine	Compazine	Involuntary movement of face or limbs, fatigue, dry mouth, blurred vision, dizziness

III. Preventive medications		
Antidepressants		
Nortriptyline	Pamelor	Avoid with MAO inhibitor; may lead to nausea, dizziness, drowsiness, blurred vision, dry mouth, weight gain; avoid with glaucoma or urinary retention
Amitriptyline	Elavil, Endep	
Doxepin	Sinequan	
Fluoxetine	Prozac	Anxiety, insomnia or drowsiness, dizziness, tremor, sweating; avoid with MAO inhibitor
Beta-blockers		
Propranolol	Inderal	Avoid with asthma, heart disease, or depression, or if diabetic on insulin; may lead to dizziness
Nadolol	Corgard	
Atenolol	Tenormin	
Timolol	Blocadren	
Calcium channel blockers		
Verapamil	Isoptin, Calan	Avoid with heart disease or low blood pressure; may lead to nausea, dizziness, constipation
Nifedipine	Procardia, Adalat	May lead to heart problems, low blood pressure, nausea, dizziness, edema; may cause headache

(cont.)

TABLE 4 *(cont.)*

Generic name	Selected trade names	Cautions and possible side effects*
Calcium channel blockers *(cont.)*		
Nimodipine	Nimotop	May lead to low blood pressure, nausea; may cause headache
Diltiazem	Cardizem	Avoid with heart disease or low blood pressure; may lead to nausea, dizziness; may cause headache
MAO inhibitor		
Phenelzine	Nardil	Must follow strict tyramine-free diet; avoid with heart or liver disease; interacts with many drugs, also with alcohol; may lead to dizziness, drowsiness
Anticonvulsants		
Carbamazepine	Tegretol	Avoid with MAO inhibitor or glaucoma; may lead to dizziness, drowsiness, nausea; requires regular monitoring for severe blood disorder
Phenytoin	Dilantin	May lead to dizziness, drowsiness, enlarged gums, unstable gait
Valproic acid	Depakote	Avoid with liver disease; may lead to nausea, vomiting, drowsiness, tremor
Others		
Methysergide	Sansert	Same as ergotamine, plus avoid with phlebitis or lung disease; may lead to fiber buildup
Lithium	Lithane, Lithobid, Eskalith	May lead to tremor, nausea, drowsiness

(cont.)

TABLE 4 *(cont.)*

Generic name	Selected trade names	Cautions and possible side effects[*]
Others *(cont.)*		
Cyclobenzaprine	Flexeril	Avoid with MAO inhibitor; drowsiness, dizziness, dry mouth
Clonidine	Catapres	Effect may be reduced if taking tricyclic antidepressants; dry mouth, drowsiness
Cyproheptadine	Periactin	Avoid with glaucoma or prostate condition; may lead to drowsiness, fatigue

Note. This is not an exhaustive list of possible side effects. Complete information should be obtained from your physician.

clinic. Use this chart only as a starting point; be sure to ask your own physician for updated information on any drug before taking it.

Again, you must be a systematic observer to be an accurate observer. Use your diary to record side effects of medication in the same way you use it to note the positive effects of medication.

8. Remember That Prescriptions and Dosages Can Be Changed According to Your Individual Needs

As we have noted, prescribing for headache management is not an exact science; there are several classes of medication, many choices within each class, and a range of possible dosages. Sometimes, for reasons not well understood, a certain medication will not work for you or might even cause problems. Other medicines, even of the same type, might have to be used in trial-and-error fashion to find exactly the right medicine or combination of medicines to control your headaches. Don't be discouraged if the first choice does not prove successful. If you cannot understand the rationale behind your physician's medication choices, ask for a clear explanation. If it seems to make sense to you, the chances are better that it is a reasonable course to pursue. If you can't understand or have doubts, ask for a simpler explanation or suggest a second opinion. It should be no insult to your physician; anyone who knows this area understands how complicated it is for patient and doctor alike.

9. Insist on Open Communications

No one likes to feel like a pest, and people with chronic pain are sometimes demoralized by their dependence on medical care. Am I worrying too much? Am I failing to tell my doctors important information? These conflicting feelings can dissuade some patients from consulting their medical team when they should and lead to impulsive calls or visits to new doctors when anxiety gets too high to control. With chronic severe headache you need to establish clear ground rules for communication with your treatment team. You must have a firm understanding of when and about what it is reasonable to call, even during off hours. You need a plan for emergency care. You need regularly scheduled visits at which to bring up questions and observations from your diary. This kind of clarity, established before a crisis, will facilitate a doctor–patient relationship satisfying to you and your treatment team. In Chapter 2 we listed some questions to ask of your doctors. Here are some others to make sure the lines of communication stay open with your physician:

+ What sorts of problems warrant an immediate call, and which should I just record in my diary and report at my next appointment?
+ What should I do if I have a severe, intolerable headache? What if this occurs at night or on a weekend?
+ What is a good time to reach you when my concern is not an emergency?
+ Who else on the treatment team can speak with me about medication questions or medical symptoms when you are unavailable?
+ Who is available when you are on vacation? Are there special rules I should know for reaching that person?
+ How often will we have regularly scheduled appointments?

When you feel free to consult your physician about your medication or your symptoms, you're less likely to make ill-advised decisions on your own, decisions that can lead to unfortunate interactions with your headache medication or wasted time and money in inadvisable treatments.

10. Avoid Self-Prescribing and Experimenting with Medications

Another unwise use of medication occurs when you deviate from your physician's instructions for its use. It is also poor judgment to supplement your prescriptions for headache control without your doctor's advice or approval. Too often headache patients see medication as the only treatment and their physician as just one source of medicine. In this lopsided view, some headache patients use over-the-counter medications, borrowed prescription medication, prescriptions from other physicians, or any number of other nontraditional medication remedies without coordinating the whole regimen through their physician.

You must realize that most of what you put in your mouth in the form of treatment for headache, natural or synthetic, has some effect on your body and on other medicines. Taking additional medications without consulting your doctor can result in a variety of adverse effects, including unexpected side effects, reduced therapeutic effects, overdose, or even aggravation of the headache syndrome. The results could be dangerous: sedation or mental confusion, cardiovascular changes such as lowered blood pressure or cardiac arrythmia, or stomach ulcers. Reduced flow of blood to certain areas of the body can damage the heart, kidneys, brain, lungs, or extremities such as fingertips.

Think of your physician as the coordinator for all medicines ingested. Before using a new medicine or other ingested remedy, talk it over and consider the possible results, positive and negative. If for any reason you are nervous about talking with your physician about medications he or she has not prescribed, or about natural remedies or any other therapy you may have heard of, bring up this nervousness at your next visit. At worst, if you really are treated rudely, you will know it is time to seek another physician.

The Goal: Simplify Your Medication

Overall, one goal of the comprehensive headache clinic is to simplify your medication regimen. Your physician will try to select medications carefully so that you are able to gain effective control with fewer types of medication. The rest of your treatment team will try to introduce other nonmedication therapies so that you will have to use less of the medications available to you. The whole goal of treatment is to help you take control of headaches so that eventually you will have to use medications only once in a while, for the severe headache that breaks through in the presence of a major trigger.

There are many advantages to reducing your reliance on medication for headache control. First, the medication that you do use will be more effective. Second, there is less risk of undesired damage to other organs of your body. Third, you are more in touch with your body and the impact of your behavior on your health. To be in touch with the impact of your behavior on your own health is not only to take on a responsibility; there is a sense of reasonable control as well, which can be very positive. You might think of it as like driving a sports car compared with a large touring sedan. In neither case do you do it alone; you need a knowledgeable team to keep the car going. But in that sports car the feel of the road can be quite exhilarating. You really feel you are driving.

One of the hardest times to face medication changes is when your treatment team, usually at the time of your initial evaluation, comes to the conclusion that your current medication regimen actually is hurting you more than it's helping. It may be very difficult to consider withdrawing from medication that has seemed to be your only hope. The withdrawal from very frequent use of painkillers or certain types of abortive medication can be painful. However, as you will see in the rest of this chapter, there are effective medication regimens that do not rely on daily or near-daily use of such medicines. These medication regimens are made more effective when combined with the other modes of treatment described in the following chapters.

MEDICATION FOR MIGRAINE HEADACHES

Your physician may prescribe *symptomatic* or *preventive* medication if your headaches are diagnosed as migraine. Symptomatic medication may be *abortive* or *analgesic*. Abortive medications are intended to stop a headache once it has begun. Analgesic medications primarily reduce or eliminate pain. Analgesic medications may also stop the headache by eliminating the pain and/or allowing sleep for a sufficient period of time. Most, but not all, symptomatic medications are more effective against migraine when taken early in the attack. However, they are not meant to be taken preventively. That practice, usually born of fear and anxiety, can lead to excessive use of abortive or analgesic medications.

Preventive or *prophylactic* medications, on the other hand, are meant to be taken daily regardless of whether or not you have a headache. These medicines are intended to modify conditions in your body to reduce the chance of migraine attacks occurring in the first place.

Your physician will determine what combination of symptomatic and preventive medication to use, based in part on the frequency of your headaches. Most physicians will prescribe only abortive and/or analgesic medication for headaches that occur once a month or less. If you are having migraines twice a month or more often, especially if they are in combination with tension-type headaches or chronic local pain, preventive medication probably will be prescribed in addition to avoid too-frequent use of analgesic or abortive medications, which is associated with rebound headache, discussed later in this chapter. Symptomatic medications should usually be limited to two days per week.

The following discussion of some of the more common medications that you may be given after evaluation for headaches is not meant to be exhaustive and is no substitute for a thorough discussion with your physician prior to using any medicine.

Abortive and Analgesic Medications

Ergotamine derivatives, made from a fungus that grows on rye, are the earliest form of abortive medications for migraine and have been one of the most commonly used. Ergotamine is a potent constrictor of arteries. Important for headache control, it constricts the arteries outside the skull, reducing the throbbing pain of migraine. However, there are several other effects of ergot derivatives that may be equally or more important in the control of migraine. Whatever the mechanism, it is an effective agent for many people. The greatest caution is that its use must be limited to two days per week to be sure of avoiding rebound headache. In addition, your physician will set an overall limit of the number of doses to be used per day or per week. As with any medication, there are also contraindications to its use with certain medical conditions, all of which must be considered individually with your physician. Ergotamine derivatives come in several forms. In addition to oral preparations, they can be received as suppositories or by needle. The latter, known as *DHE-45,* is often used intravenously as an abortive agent when a migraine headache is both severe and prolonged. This kind of treatment is often given in an emergency room.

The newest abortive medication is *sumatriptan,* which promotes vasoconstriction as do the ergot derivatives. It is effective in reducing the severe pain of migraine to mild or no pain in about 70 percent of patients. However, it also has side effects, and its use must be restricted in some persons, particularly those with any symptoms of cardiovascular disease. At present, sumatriptan is available in kits that allow you to inject yourself, under the skin, without an elaborate procedure. It is expensive, but compared with a visit to the emergency room the cost is quite reasonable.

Used as part of an overall plan for control of migraine, it has already proven to be an important part of the "tool box." In the future, oral and suppository forms of sumatriptan may be available in the United States.

Another form of abortive medication has the intimidating name *isometheptene*. The most common brand name with this medication is Midrin, which also contains acetaminophen and dichloralphenazone, another tongue twister. This is an important medication for migraine patients who cannot use sumatriptan or ergot derivatives.

Analgesics come in many types and combinations. It would be prohibitive to try to name every analgesic you might find, from your physician or over the counter. They are also heavily advertised, to professionals and to the public. Here we will try only to summarize the most common forms and combinations and repeat the general caution not to fall into the trap of overusing such medications.

Aspirin and acetaminophen are the most common analgesics. They may be prescribed alone or in combination with caffeine, barbiturates, or narcotics. Aspirin and acetaminophen are sometimes dismissed by headache sufferers as less powerful because they are so accessible. In fact, however, they are potent painkillers, and it was not long ago that aspirin was considered the wonder drug of its age. These analgesics have a place in the treatment of mild to moderate headache and must not be overused, to avoid organ damage or the risk of rebound headache. In combination with caffeine, absorption of the analgesic is improved, putting it to work more quickly. Caffeine also constricts blood vessels temporarily and may have its own analgesic effect. Used no more than two days per week, this combination can be useful. The great risk for the headache patient is that the addition of caffeine to the analgesic (when used more frequently than two days a week) can make rebound headache more likely. The addition of barbiturates to a compound gives a sedating effect, which can promote sleep and calming. Barbiturates are one of the higher risks for overuse and dependence, thus leading to rebound headache. Similar cautions apply to the many analgesic compounds with narcotic medication (see, for example, those listed in Table 4).

Nonsteroidal anti-inflammatory (NSAI) medications are becoming commonplace among the analgesic medications. Several types are now available in over-the-counter preparations. Ibuprofen is perhaps the best known. They are generally used as symptomatic medications but can be useful for prevention of some types of headaches, especially migraines that occur regularly with the menstrual cycle. There are many similarities to aspirin in the mechanisms of action and side effects. As with all analgesic medications, frequent use carries with it risk for rebound head-ache and organ damage. Stomach irritation is not an unusual problem with frequent use of aspirin or NSAI medication.

Preventive Medications for Chronic Migraine

Preventive medications are used when migraine headaches have become as frequent as twice a month and you've had limited success in treating the particular attacks. As migraine headaches come more frequently, there is greater risk of tension-type headache as well. The more days of some type of headache, the more risk there is of excessive use of abortive or analgesic medication.

Preventive medications are found to be less effective when there is overuse of symptomatic medications. It is important, especially if pre-ventive medication is being introduced only after headache has become very frequent (fifteen or more headache days per month), that sympto-matic medication be reduced as preventive medication is being started. However, preventive medications do not preclude the use of sympto-matic medication; it is common to have an abortive medication for use with severe headache that breaks through. Nevertheless, it is important to limit the frequency of symptomatic medication. At the very least, even when it is necessary for a time to use symptomatic medication on a daily basis, your headache specialist is likely to ask you to take it at regular times rather than whenever you think you need it. As with all medication regimens for chronic severe headache, it is also critical that it be part of a comprehensive treatment plan, using nonmedication therapies as well.

There are many different types of preventive drugs. Again, the sheer variety of medications makes it impossible for us to offer an exhaustive discussion of them. The choice of appropriate preventive medications rests with your physician. Effects may not be evident for several weeks, so patience is required in finding the right preventive medication.

The following drugs do have a preventive effect against migraines, but keep in mind that they are not cures. You may still have migraines, but if you use your medication wisely, they will probably be less frequent, less intense, and shorter. It's important to take them in the proper dose at the proper time every day, whether or not you have a headache.

For near-daily headaches, *antidepressant* medications are probably the most commonly prescribed preventive medicine. Although devel-oped initially to treat depression, these medicines have been found to be extremely effective in the treatment of chronic pain conditions of many types. In the 1970s, controlled studies demonstrated that one of the early antidepressants, *amitriptyline,* was effective in reducing headache frequency. Although pain, depression, and sleep experiences seem to be related, the effect on headaches was not due primarily to the effect of the medicine on depression. Amitriptyline is called a *tricyclic* antidepressant, reflecting its chemical makeup. There are other types, closely related, which are used to avoid some of the side effects of amitriptyline, although they have not been studied as extensively. New forms of antidepressant medications, more selective in their effect on a particular chemical called *serotonin,* have also been used in prevention of headache. In general these medications have fewer side effects than the tricyclic antidepressants. Fluoxetine (Prozac) is the drug of this type most commonly recognized by the public.

Beta-adrenergic blockers may be the most common preventive for migraine headache that is not occurring on a near-daily basis. Clinically, we have not found them to be as effective as antidepressant medication for very frequent severe headaches. There are several types of beta-adrenergic medicines effective with migraine in research studies, and propanolol (Inderal) may be the most commonly recognized by the public. Its effectiveness with migraine was discovered accidentally in the 1960s and was confirmed in later controlled studies. Like antidepressant medication, there are several mechanisms of action that may contribute to the effectiveness of beta-adrenergic blockers in headaches. Part of the effect may be due to the blocking of the beta-adrenergic receptors, which prevents vasodilation. As with all medications, there are side effects and interactions with other medications and diseases. The choice of medication—among beta-adrenergic blockers, among preventive medications in general, and among all possible medications in headache management—is a complicated decision that rests ultimately in the hands of your physician.

Many other preventive medication regimens may be used, a number of them listed in Table 4 but only a few discussed here. Many are treated in more detail in books more oriented toward medication management (see "Further Reading" at the back of this book). Your physician can also copy descriptions of particular medicines he or she wishes to consider with you from more technical books available to the headache specialist.

Among the other preventive medications, *monoamine oxidase (MAO) inhibitors* are used often for patients with migraine headaches not responding to other treatments. These medications require the patient to follow a special diet before, during, and after treatment. Foods containing tyramine (see the section on headache and diet in Chapter 5), alcohol, and caffeine are especially problematic. There are also strict limitations on the use of some other drugs.

Calcium channel antagonists (blockers) are a mixed group of medicines that are not as commonly used as the beta-adrenergic blockers in the treatment of migraine. However, they are often tried when a person cannot use a beta-blocker because of other medical conditions. The way in which these drugs affect migraine is not known for certain; as with the other preventive medications, several mechanisms of action may be important.

Methysergide (Sansert), closely related chemically to the ergot derivatives, prevents migraines but also has serious side effects if used for too long. It can establish a prolonged state of vasoconstriction, with the buildup of fibrous tissue affecting the heart, kidneys, and other organs. Based on current knowledge, it is wise not to take methysergide for longer than six months without a six- to eight-week break. The patient who is using methysergide should have regular medical evaluations to avoid dangerous complications.

A Special Challenge:
The Transition to Preventive Medication

Over time most people with migraine notice that headache frequency increases and decreases according to current psychological or social stressors, changes in diet or medication, health changes, and a variety of other factors, recognized or not. Many reach a point at which their headache frequency increases and then does not improve. This is often when headache sufferers go through a number of health care providers, trying various treatments. At some point in this difficult course they may be referred to a comprehensive headache treatment center.

In the initial evaluation of a person with frequent headaches, it is not unusual to find that symptomatic medication use (analgesic and/or abortive) is just as frequent as the headaches. For that reason it is likely that the physician will recommend a transition from reliance on symptomatic medication to preventive medication. For optimal effect of the preventive medication, if you find yourself in this situation, you must be prepared to withdraw from (reduce markedly) the symptomatic medication.

This transition from symptomatic to preventive medication can be difficult, especially if you have been using symptomatic medication on many days (more than two days per week is considered high). If your symptomatic medication has included a compound with barbiturates, caffeine, or narcotics, you may have pain or other symptoms during the time of withdrawal. The anxiety that often accompanies reduction in symptomatic medication makes the process even more discomfiting.

These challenging circumstances may tempt you to do exactly the wrong thing: stop the process of withdrawal and return to the symptomatic medication. It is important that you stay the course. Learn from your treatment team what to expect during withdrawal so you won't be caught off guard. Ask your physician what kind of medication assistance you can expect to ease the discomfort. Use behavioral techniques with your biobehavioral therapist to calm your anxiety and relax your body so you won't experience even worse pain. If you can get past the first few days, you are on the way toward taking control of headache. If you return to overuse of symptomatic medication, it is the drug that is in control, creating headaches as it wears off.

Reactions to withdrawal and ability to work with pain vary widely from individual to individual. You may be one of those whose transition can be managed at home with medical supervision. Even here you may be well advised to take a few days away from your regular routine, taking time off work and/or getting assistance for domestic responsibilities. Make arrangements with your treatment team, family, and friends for behavioral support. Others, however, suffer intolerable pain, vomiting, and emotional distress. This reaction to withdrawal is no reflection on your character or strength. It simply means that you will require closer monitoring, medication assistance, and psychological support, which can be accomplished most effectively as a hospital inpatient.

MEDICATION
FOR TENSION-TYPE HEADACHES

The basic principle for medication treatment of tension-type headaches is similar to that for migraines: infrequent headaches call for symptomatic medication, and more frequent ones call for preventive. In most cases of *intermittent* (or episodic) tension headaches—often occurring less than once a week—medication is simple and nonproblematic. Generally, simple analgesics—aspirin, acetaminophen, or nonsteroidal anti-inflammatory medication—will suffice. Sometimes caffeine is added to the analgesic to improve absorption in the stomach, leading to more effective relief. These medications usually will abort the headache, not just dull the pain.

When tension headaches become more frequent, especially when they occur 15 days a month or more, it is no longer practical to use symptomatic medication. The problem is the same as when migraine headache develops into daily or near-daily headache; use of symptomatic medication under these conditions markedly increases the risk of rebound headache. Unsystematic use of the analgesic—using it without a strict timetable—seems to increase the problem. Caffeine, an effective agent with analgesic medication when used sparingly, seems to further increase the risk of rebound headache when used more than two or three days per week. The problem with caffeine is only compounded by other sources of caffeine in your daily diet—coffee, tea, and cola being the most common.

At this point your physician usually will suggest that multimodal treatment is necessary for comprehensive treatment of the headache. For the medication part of treatment he or she is likely to suggest relying primarily on preventive medication, usually an antidepressant. Most often the tricyclic antidepressants are used, particularly if you're having difficulty with sleep. When these medications are taken prior to sleep, they cause fewer problems with sedation as a side effect, and they help you get to sleep and sleep well. Using this medication to accomplish both goals also keeps the medication plan just that much simpler. If you have been using analgesic medication very frequently, you may go through a period of increased headache and other discomfort as you withdraw from the analgesic medication. As with their use in chronic daily headache that has developed from migraine, the antidepressants are prescribed to be taken each day, in a specific dose, at specific times. Normally you will continue to use this medication for at least six months.

Research is not yet clear on the subject, but tension-type headaches are likely to be found to be a less severe variant of migraine. Many trigger factors can promote tension headaches, but depression and psychological stress are very common. Although stress is very often present, tranquilizers are not often part of the medication plan in a comprehensive headache clinic. There are many potential problems with regular use of tranquilizers, and they do not usually add very much to what other medications, more effective for headache treatment, can offer. Too often in our experience tranquilizers become a crutch that is hard to give up. Biobehavioral therapy may seem like more trouble than "popping" another pill, but we recommend you think twice before starting to take tranquilizers for headache management. Biobehavioral therapy is a much safer addition to the multimodal treatment plan for chronic tension-type headache. What you learn can become part of your life for a long time, improving its quality beyond the effect on headaches.

MEDICATION FOR CLUSTER HEADACHES

As with tension and migraine headaches, the approach to medication treatment for cluster headaches varies with the frequency of the headache. However, the nature of cluster headaches requires that we look at frequency somewhat differently. As suggested by their name, cluster headaches occur in bunches. Each headache is relatively brief, but they occur one or more times per day for days, weeks, or months at a time. In episodic cluster headache there are periods of no headache that may last for weeks, months, or even years. In chronic cluster headache these periods of respite become shorter or nonexistent.

Episodic Cluster Headache

Because the duration of each individual headache is short, the major goal of medication treatment is to stop the cluster. Treatment for each individual headache (abortive medication) may be given, but it is not the primary focus. Abortive medication may include use of ergotamine derivatives in various forms, sumatriptan, or oxygen inhalation. Preventive medication is started as soon as possible after a cluster begins. *Steroids* are very effective for cluster headache, especially when the clusters are separated by long periods of respite. They are not without risk, and their use is limited carefully. Steroids are prescribed usually for a two-week period only, in declining doses. They are not appropriate for chronic use.

Chronic Cluster Headache

Chronic cluster headache is a special case. When the severe pain of cluster headaches does not respond to the usual medication to end the cluster, and when the typical periods of respite seem to vanish, extended use of preventive medications may be required. *Verapamil,* a calcium channel antagonist, is a commonly used medication for chronic cluster headache. Other medications that might be considered include *methysergide, ergot derivatives,* and *lithium.* Each is taken at specified times and in fixed dosages. As with any medicine used for a longer period of time, great attention must be given to medical monitoring to detect any adverse effects of these medications as early as possible. Each medicine carries its own risks, and you should ask to be made aware of them before starting and while you continue to use the medicine. In this way you can help your team balance benefits and risks in a healthy way.

Several headache syndromes, which may be variants of cluster headache, are distinguished by their response to a *nonsteroidal anti-inflammatory* drug called *indomethacin*. The most well-known of these syndromes may be *paroxysmal hemicrania*. This variant affects women more than men, as opposed to cluster headache, which affects mostly men. The pain of paroxysmal hemicrania is very brief but also very frequent. Cluster headache and these variants are much less common than migraine or tension headaches.

MEDICATION-INDUCED HEADACHE

The focus of this chapter has been two-fold: to give you some basic information about some medications used to treat the most common headache types and to help you understand the role of medication as part of a comprehensive treatment plan for frequent severe headaches. With regard to the former, it is important not to equate reading this chapter with having received a medical education. While we believe that it is vital for you to be an informed member of the treatment team, we also remind you that prescribing for headache management involves a complex series of judgments having to do not only with the headache itself but with your overall health and any other medications you may be taking. Your active role in this process involves asking questions until you understand, reporting positive and negative effects of the medication, and bringing your own ideas to the consulting room for discussion. The physician's role is still to *lead* the treatment team in its consideration of the medication portion of the comprehensive treatment plan.

The second focus—to understand the role of medication as *part* of the comprehensive treatment plan for frequent severe headaches—is just as important. Medication cannot do the whole job in most cases of frequent severe headaches. In such cases trying to use medication as the whole treatment plan leads to a frustrating series of ineffective medication trials over months of wasted time. In the worst cases overuse of medication can result in serious side effects or can even make the headache syndrome worse. While overuse of compounds containing barbiturates and ergotamine is of greatest concern, overuse of even simple over-the-counter analgesics such as aspirin, acetaminophen, or ibuprofen can lead to this type of rebound or drug-induced headache in those who have intermittent headache syndromes. The drug overuse actually seems to overpower even the intended effect of preventive medications. The exact mechanism (and there may be more than one) by which overuse of medication makes headache syndromes worse is not entirely clear, but we have seen over and over again that for most patients, by far, withdrawal from overuse of abortive and analgesic medications decreases the frequency and duration of the headaches.

How can you tell whether you may have medication-induced headache? First, of course, you will be having headache, sometimes with mixed symptoms of migraine and tension headaches, very often, fifteen or more days per month. You are using medication, perhaps a lot of it, but it doesn't seem to help. If it does help, the benefit wears off after a short time. Second, you will be using symptomatic medication very often. Even if the medication does not seem to be helping, you continue to use it for fear the headache will just be worse if you did not take it. When you are using analgesic or abortive medication more than two days a week, the risk of rebound headache is increased. Third, you may notice that you are requiring a higher dosage of your usual medication to get the same effect. There can be a gradual escalation of medication doses because your body has gotten used to having this medication. Fourth, you begin to use symptomatic medications preventively. That is, you use them before you have symptoms because you are afraid they will develop. Fifth, a growing tension between you and your physician can be a sign that you are beginning to demand medication and that your physician is becoming conflicted between wanting to help and worrying about your increasing reliance on medication.

If you recognize any of these signs in yourself, we urge you to seek help in simplifying your medication. Obviously this is a hard step to take. If you're reading this book because you are about to consult a headache specialist at a comprehensive headache center, you'll find expert help there. If you're still working only with your primary care physician, broach this subject. He or she is undoubtedly just as frustrated as you are with the failure to progress toward controlling your headaches. Express your willingness to reconsider your medication regimen and to try other modes of therapy at the same time. Your physician is very likely to welcome your openness to developing a more comprehensive treatment plan with the consultation of other headache specialists.

✦ THE CASE OF KAREN L., PART 3

Karen's physician advised her to continue taking the antidepressant
medication each night, but many of the other medication changes
turned in the direction of reduction and simplification. She was
asked to discontinue the prescribed and over-the-counter analgesic
medications. A new nonsteroidal anti-inflammatory medication
was introduced, taken regularly three times per day. During the first
week of reducing the analgesic medication, Karen made specific
plans with her physician about what she should do if a severe
headache broke through. They included an abortive medication in
addition to other nonmedication coping strategies developed with
the psychologist and biobehavioral therapist, with strict limits on
how often the abortive medication could be used. There was also a
backup plan to call the physician if headache pain was intolerable.
She was referred to a sinus and allergy specialist for an opinion about
her chronic congestion; the specialist was asked to make a diagnosis
and to give Karen the simplest form of treatment that would still give
relief from the congestion. The estrogen supplement was considered
necessary by her gynecologist, but the lowest possible necessary
dose was agreed on by the headache team physician and gynecologist. They agreed to review the results and consider other forms of
estrogen in the future if necessary.

Karen got immediate results from simplifying her medication.
Within two weeks her headaches decreased in severity. By the third
week she noticed a day or two without headache at all. In retrospect
it seemed clear that Karen's use of medication had increased, rather
than eased, her headaches. Simplifying it was a first step toward
taking control.

Karen's physical and biobehavioral therapy are discussed in the
following chapters. Here we can look ahead far enough to say that
after two months of this combination of therapies Karen reported
remarkable improvement. The nonsteroidal anti-inflammatory
medication was reduced to twice per day, and Karen was having to
use the abortive medication much less often. She continued on the
antidepressant medication. At about this time Karen's physical therapy ended, but her biobehavioral therapy continued. At the end of
three months of treatment Karen had taken enough control of her
headaches that her physician recommended further reduction in
medication. He suggested that Karen gradually taper and eliminate

regular use of the nonsteroidal anti-inflammatory. The amitriptyline was continued.

The goal of the physician in Karen's case, as part of the comprehensive treatment team, was to use the least medication necessary to help control the headache. This involves wise choices of the type of medication to be used and the types of medication to be discontinued. It also involves wise choices about the way the selected medication is used—dosages, schedules, and forms in which it is administered. Once the headache is initially under control, some types of medication can be phased out of regular use. Others are continued for a longer time. Karen is cautioned that the headache syndrome has been managed, not cured, and is urged to continue to use what she has learned in her biobehavioral and physical therapies in some form that she can incorporate into her lifestyle. We will discuss these therapies in the chapters that follow, where we will continue Karen's story.

✦

CHAPTER 7

Relieve Muscle Tension: Physical Therapy

I n physical therapy you learn about the workings and condition of your muscles and joints, receive in-office treatments, and develop an exercise program for stretching and strengthening the muscles of the upper body to use at home. This combination of education, treatment, and home exercise regimen is known to be effective in restoring health to muscles and joints—restoring range of motion, reducing muscle tenderness and stiffness, modifying habitual postures or movements, and strengthening underused muscles—and thus in helping you take control of your headaches. The areas of greatest concern to the headache patient are the upper back, neck and face.

If you are going to a comprehensive headache clinic, the doctors on the treatment team are quite likely to recommend physical therapy as part of your treatment if they find indications of muscle irritation in the initial evaluations. Muscle irritation is often an important trigger or contributing factor in chronic severe headache of any type. It is frequently, but not always, the result of prolonged muscle tension associated with psychological stress or poor physical habits. If you've been consulting only your primary care physician, you may want to ask if he or she has considered physical therapy for you. This chapter focuses on the physical therapy evaluation and treatment you might encounter at a comprehensive headache clinic.

YOUR DOCTOR'S ROLE

At a headache clinic the decision to incorporate physical therapy into your treatment will be based on your doctors' initial evaluations of your headaches. They will look for muscle irritation by examining the range of motion of your neck, shoulders, and jaw, as well as muscle stiffness and/or tenderness at the upper back, neck, and face.

Range of motion is assessed by having you move these parts of your body in prescribed ways—leaning your neck to each side, moving your neck backward and forward, turning or rotating your neck to each side, opening your jaw as far as you can—as your doctor observes. You will be asked to report muscle stiffness or pain as you move. Muscle stiffness or tenderness also is determined by pressing against the muscles, feeling their texture, and asking you to report any areas of tenderness. You will be asked to report whether the tenderness you feel seems to spread out from the area that was pressed. Areas of severe pain, often with pain spreading to other parts of the upper body, are called *trigger points*. In talking with you about the history of your headaches, the physician will ask you to recall any accident in which your muscles or bones might have been injured.

Based on these evaluations, your physician will make the ultimate decision as to whether you need professional help from the physical therapist in relieving muscle irritation. When no indications of severe muscle irritation appear, you may be able to make any necessary changes in postural habits or chronic muscle tension on your own or in biobehavioral therapy only. When muscles have become quite irritated, however, with many indications of muscle shortening, pain with movement, stiffness, or tenderness, treating these muscles (and surrounding tissue) directly is often helpful.

THE FIELD OF PHYSICAL THERAPY

Physical therapy is a health specialty that began about fifty years ago to help the injured from World War II and the victims of polio epidemics. Its goal at that time was simply to get people up and walking, back to as much of their normal daily activity as possible. Since then, physical therapy has expanded into areas ranging from cardiovascular rehabilitation to sports medicine. It is offered to individuals of all ages, pediatric to geriatric, and of all levels of physical conditioning, from elite athletes to the most debilitated recoverees. Physical therapists may be found treating almost any muscle, joint, or muscle/joint combination. The goal of physical therapy today is to enhance physical rehabilitation following injury or disease or in any chronic condition.

All physical therapists must be certified by a state board. Most have at least a bachelor's degree, though the American Physical Therapy Association is now advocating a master's degree. In some states physical therapists practice only by referral; in others patients have direct access to them. In either case physical therapists may advertise their specialties as other professionals do.

As the field has expanded, individual physical therapists have begun to specialize; for that reason not all are equally qualified to treat headache-related muscle irritation. If you are not working with the treatment team of a comprehensive headache clinic, be sure that your physician helps you select a physical therapist who has specific training and experience working with chronic conditions in general and headaches in particular.

THE PHYSICAL THERAPIST'S EXAMINATION

If you have been referred to the physical therapist by your physician, the doctor will give directions regarding the desired treatment. If the physical therapist is part of your regular treatment team at the clinic, he or she will receive or have access to your complete chart. The chart will include the history of your headache and the results of x-rays, blood tests, or other diagnostic work that has been done. In either case, clear communication between the physical therapist and the other members of your treatment team, then and during the course of treatment, is essential for most effective care.

The therapist will review the initial information with you, asking especially about events or activities, even those that happened long ago, that may have injured muscle or led you to alter your normal movement or posture and thus resulted in muscle irritation. These could be major events such as injuries and diseases but may also include the little things in your daily routine—at home, at work, at leisure—that build up over time. Many jobs, for example, require you to repeat certain motions or maintain a rigid posture throughout the day, leading to fatigue and muscle tension. The physical therapist will also be attentive to evidence of psychological stress or biological changes that may lead to muscle tension and irritation.

With this history in mind, the therapist will conduct a physical evaluation. He or she will concentrate mainly on the upper body—specifically the neck, jaw, and upper back—but the assessment of posture requires attention also to the pelvis, knees, and ankles. The therapist may ask you to sit, stand, or move in certain ways and may palpate various areas as your doctors did in your initial evaluations. In addition to your active movements, the physical therapist may test your range of motion passively, moving part of your body while you relax, to further assess the functioning of certain muscles and joints.

In looking for deviations from normal posture, range of motion, or muscle condition, the therapist will pay particular attention to imbalances. Do you rest more heavily on one side as you stand or sit? Can you move your neck or some other joint farther one way than the other? Do you have an especially tight or sore muscle? If an imbalance is identified, the therapist will look for its source—a joint out of alignment, shortened muscle fibers, a weakened muscle, and the like. These examples are not all that the physical therapist may try to learn in the initial examination, but they will give you an idea of some of the main things he or she hopes to learn in meeting you for the first few times.

THE PHYSICAL THERAPIST'S TREATMENT

Based on the initial medical and psychological examinations, the history of your condition, and the results of the physical therapy evaluation, your physical therapist will develop a treatment plan to help you reduce muscle irritation. Tailored to your individual condition just as a prescription for medication is, your treatment will probably be divided into three segments—education, in-office treatment, and at-home exercise—each with its own goals.

Education

The physical therapist will want to educate you about your condition, what is contributing to it, and, most important, what changes you can make to improve it. The goal is to prepare you to sustain those changes for a lifetime. Throughout this book we emphasize that headache is managed, not cured. You can easily lose the gains made if you return to the old habits that led to or maintained your muscle irritation and in the process increase the risk that headaches will return. On the other hand, if you remember the knowledge that your physical therapist imparts and keep up healthy physical habits, you have a good chance of keeping control over your headaches for a long time.

From the information gathered during the evaluation, your therapist should have a good idea of whether factors in your work or home routine—or both—are causing muscle tension. The therapist may want to visit your workplace to get a full understanding of the physical demands of your job. Domestic work and jobs outside the home can lead to muscle irritation in many ways. Desk work may not seem too physically demanding, but any kind of desk work may involve postures that can lead to imbalances in muscle and joint function. Computer operators, secretaries, executives—all those who are on the phone a lot or use office machines for extended periods—are susceptible to muscle tension and irritation. Jobs that require you to stand relatively still for long periods—assembly-line workers, hairstylists, barbers, cashiers—are also physically demanding.

After narrowing down the possible contributing factors, your therapist will suggest changes in your work routine that could be of long-term benefit. You may be advised to raise or lower a desk or other work surface, use a different kind of chair or tool, change the way you grasp or move objects, stand or sit in a more balanced position, or move around more frequently during the workday.

Housework, child care, even hobbies and recreational activities may involve motions and postures just as tension-producing as those in the workplace. Your physical therapist may suggest a different way of carrying or picking up a child, different seating for an activity such as needlework, model building, or reading, or even a different movement pattern for sweeping the floor or doing the dishes.

In-Office Treatment

The goal of in-office treatment is to help you break the pain cycle. The initial injury or prolonged tension may have irritated a specific muscle or joint. Over time, tension builds in surrounding muscles as they brace against the pain or compensate for reduced function in the painful part. The injured muscle or other muscles opposite the overused muscles may become weak from underuse. Both chronic tension and underuse, or reduced function, eventually lead to shortening of the muscle fibers. Such muscles are even more susceptible to spasm, which in turn becomes a source of pain beginning the cycle anew. In this way pain that begins in one place can spread gradually to other parts of the body. You may feel tightness in one area today, then notice similar stiffness or pain in another area tomorrow. As the areas of muscle irritation expand, the overall risk of headaches triggered by muscle irritation increases as well.

Physical therapists have at their disposal a number of passive techniques (things the therapist does to you) for breaking the pain cycle in the office. These techniques are called *modalities*. One modality a therapist may choose for you is manual therapy, including deep massage, stretching, and mobilization or movement of joints. Other modalities include treatment with heat or ice packs, ultrasound devices, and electrical stimulation, possibly with a TENS (transcutaneous, or through-the-skin, electrical nerve stimulation) unit. Whatever the modalities of choice, a good therapist will explain thoroughly how they work and how they are expected to help you.

At-Home Exercise

A competent physical therapist also knows that, in the case of chronic severe headache, in-office treatment can't do it all. You must also have an active program of stretching and strengthening exercises that you can practice in the office and carry out at home. The goal of therapeutic exercise is to stretch the shortened muscles, relaxing them physically, and to strengthen muscles that have become weak through underuse. In this way the pain cycle is also further interrupted, making your muscles more resilient and resistant to irritation. The ultimate goal is for you to continue to use these exercises to maintain reduced muscle tension on your own, even after you have stopped active physical therapy. By using them regularly, you maintain the health of your muscles and decrease the risk of headaches triggered by muscle irritation. A good stretching and strengthening regimen sometimes can bail you out even if you forgot to work actively on reducing muscle tension from psychological stress or poor postures that day.

How rapidly your therapist introduces the active exercise regimen depends in part on the condition of your muscles when you come in. Severely irritated muscles require gentle care in the beginning. It is easy to overdo the stretching and strengthening, causing muscle inflammation and pain. The resulting pain can discourage you from trying again. However, the exercise regimen is critically important, and it is often introduced early in treatment. If your muscles are very irritated, the physical therapist may start with modalities to relax the muscle before starting the exercises. At first the exercise regimen may be kept simple, with limited demand on the muscles and joints. The therapist will demonstrate the exercises for you and then watch as you try them. Based on this observation, the therapist will correct your performance of the exercise and possibly adapt the exercise to your needs or even suggest a different exercise. Through this process your exercise program becomes custom tailored.

Even with experience and due care, it is not hard to overdo exercise with severely irritated muscles. If this happens, you will experience increased pain locally, and a headache may be triggered. You may notice muscle swelling, hot sensation in the painful area, and limited range of motion. Be sure to call your physical therapist should this happen. He or she can suggest some ways to reduce the pain and swelling, like ice applied in a towel or bag to protect your skin. In addition, you will both know two things: you have discovered an area in which you must proceed slowly and cautiously, but also an area that you absolutely must address in treatment if you are to succeed in reducing the risk of headache.

In taking on responsibility for maintaining an active home exercise program, your involvement in your headache treatment plan reaches a new level of active participation. To this point you've had to be a good consumer of medical services, a diligent recordkeeper, collaborative with the professionals dedicated to helping you. Now you must actively follow through on your exercise program, faithfully doing the exercises as and when suggested. This, obviously, requires more effort than taking your medication as directed and reporting any side effects. But the rewards are ample: if you stay with them, the exercises prescribed by your physical therapist will not only reduce muscle irritation but also improve your general health.

During subsequent visits your physical therapist will want to follow up on the progress of your exercise program. The therapist will watch you do the exercises again, looking for signs of improvement as well as for changes or corrections that are needed. You will build up gradually to full range of motion and more vigorous strengthening exercises. When you are able to carry out the home exercise program fully and effectively, your in-office treatments will be reduced gradually and then limited to follow-up visits for reexamination, review of your faithfulness to the home program, observation of exercises to detect incorrect methods that may have crept in, and suggestions of additional exercises that may be called for.

◆   THE CASE OF KAREN L., PART 4

In Chapter 6 we discussed how simplifying and reducing medication alleviated some of Karen's headaches, but we emphasized that the combination of medication and other therapies, among them physical therapy, was what really put Karen in control. Karen's doctors noticed in the initial evaluations that the left side of her upper back and neck was especially tender. So were the muscles at her left temple and jaw. Karen was aware that she sometimes clenched her teeth. She could move her neck the normal distances, but with pain in some of the movements, from the left side and back of her neck. Karen's doctors referred her to the physical therapist, asking for further evaluation with special attention to the left side of the upper back and neck and to the muscles involved in use of the jaw. They knew from prior work with the therapist, a regular part of the treatment team, that he would use an active treatment regimen as much as possible, with specific work in stretching and strengthening these areas.

The physical therapist's initial evaluation found, in addition, that Karen routinely held her head in a slightly forward position. This increased the demand on the muscles of the neck. The therapist noticed also that she kept her left shoulder higher than the right and that the left trapezius, between the shoulder and the neck, was painful and would tense if pressed or squeezed lightly. Accordingly, on Karen's first visit, the therapist used modalities to relax the muscles in the areas of the left shoulder and back of the neck. One was manual stretching of the left trapezius, with the aid of an ultracoolant spray to reduce spasming. This technique is known as *spray and stretch.* After also stretching the muscles at the back of Karen's neck, the therapist applied moist heat to her left shoulder area for twenty minutes. To conclude the session, the physical therapist taught Karen three exercises that she did in the office. One was a lateral (side-to-side) stretch of the neck, one a stretch of the levator scapula muscle between the shoulder blade and the spine, and one an overhead lifting of the arms. Karen received a sheet of written instructions with a diagram for each exercise and was instructed to do them at home each day.

Karen went to physical therapy every two or three days for several weeks. The modalities were continued at each session. The therapist added deep pressure massage, transcutaneous electrical nerve stimulation (TENS), and ultrasound modalities for the left trapezius. At each session Karen would demonstrate that she remembered and could perform her home exercises correctly. She continued to do the exercises daily at home.

By the end of this active phase of treatment, Karen reported much less frequent and intense headaches. At the session that happened to mark one month since she had started physical therapy, she was pleased to be able to say that she had no headache. The physical therapist found that her upper body posture and neck range of motion were improved significantly. The muscles at the upper back, neck, and face were much less tender, so much so that the therapist felt she could go a few weeks without further sessions. The combination of in-office treatment and the home exercise regimen had helped Karen reduce the muscle irritation that had been a significant factor leading to her more frequent headaches.

At a follow-up session three weeks later Karen reported only a few headaches. Most important for the goals of the physical therapist, she demonstrated no unusual muscle tenderness and normal movement at the upper body. Her therapist recommended no further sessions but urged Karen to maintain the home exercises that were so obviously helping to control her headaches. The therapist also recommended that Karen begin a walking program to enhance her overall health.

Muscle irritation and the muscle tension that is so often a cause of the irritation are important factors in many cases of chronic severe headache. We presume that a person must have a propensity to headache for the muscle irritation to trigger headaches; certainly we have seen people with significant upper-body muscle irritation who report only local pain at the neck or head. However, in a person who is prone to headache, muscle irritation is important to consider among the many factors that can make headaches more frequent. In people with frequent severe headache, muscle irritation is very common and may be involved in a vicious circle with the headache leading to more muscle tension and the tension leading to muscle irritation and more headache. Among people who have had some type of accident, even if it did not seem to be very severe, it is not unusual to find muscle irritation at the neck or jaw that seems to play an important role in causing and maintaining headache.

The prospect of reducing muscle irritation is well worth your effort in keeping up the home exercise program. The combination of patient education, in-office treatment, and at-home exercise offered through the physical therapist is a powerful ally as you continue to take control of your headaches. It's not your only ally, however. Keep in mind that as Karen reduced her medication and participated in physical therapy, she was undergoing other therapies concurrently. These are described in the following chapters.

✦

CHAPTER 8

Reduce Internal Tension: Relaxation in the Control of Headaches

I nternal tension is one of the final common pathways to chronic and severe headaches. It can trigger headaches and contribute to an "internal environment" that makes headaches more likely to occur with other triggers, as described in Chapter 4. The significant role of internal tension makes relaxation therapy one of the most important modes of treatment for controlling headaches. In some form relaxation training is likely to be part of any multimodal treatment plan in a comprehensive headache clinic. This chapter explains the many ways in which relaxation training helps to reduce internal tension and how it fits into biobehavioral treatment in general.

There are many different ways to learn relaxation of mind and body. You might think of these different methods as different roads to the same place. The form that is used depends on many things, including which ones your treatment team is familiar with, but your comfort and preference are not small factors in the final choice. Naturally the method chosen must also be effective at achieving relaxation of physical systems like muscle and nervous system activity, which can be measured in the office. In the following pages we describe the most common relaxation methods to introduce you to some of the available options. Effective relaxation training requires practice and attention to your body. It is not a technique to be done mechanically or sloppily. Most often you will benefit from learning relaxation with a biobehavioral therapist to help you refine your technique, provide physical measurement to ensure that it is having the desired effect, and add behavior therapy to help you actually use the relaxation in changing your everyday life. However, this chapter provides enough detail to serve as a supplement to the information and experience you will receive from your therapist. You will also find here clinical hints drawn from our experience that may make the relaxation techniques more effective for you. Consider using this chapter as a periodic review while you're learning relaxation.

As important as it is, remember that relaxation is still only one mode of treatment—no more the single cure or "fix" for your chronic headache than medication or physical therapy. Long-term resolution of your problem is much more likely with patient use of several reliable forms of therapy simultaneously, under the direction of an experienced treatment team. Relaxation training will augment the effectiveness of the other therapies, and they will augment the effectiveness of relaxation training. Relaxation training is further augmented by the use of biofeedback. Undertaken in the context of biobehavioral therapy, the beneficial effects of relaxation can extend far beyond the walls of your therapist's office and into your entire life. Finally, as you learn to identify recurring sources of internal tension in your life, you will have taken the first step toward changing them as well.

THE GOAL OF RELAXATION THERAPY

Internal tension can also be described as stress. As mentioned in Chapter 4, stress comes in welcome and unwelcome forms. It can, in fact, be defined as anything that we perceive as a challenge. This challenge may come with the excitement of being the guest of honor at a birthday party thrown by family and friends or making the trade of a lifetime on the floor of the commodities exchange; it may appear in the threat of losing an important contract to a rival or driving your family through a blizzard. Whatever the experience, the body reacts with arousal, gearing up to meet the demands of the situation. In such situations you may notice a variety of physical responses. Your hands or feet may become cool and damp; your face or neck may flush and feel hot. Your breathing may become more shallow and rapid, with a corresponding increase in the strength and speed of the heartbeat. Muscles of the neck and face may contract. Emotional intensity may increase, leading you to speak or act in ways that you hope will resolve the threat. Other effects, such as elevated blood pressure, dilation of pupils, and release of certain hormones into the bloodstream, are less noticeable to us but still may be significant for your headache.

Sometimes this arousal is called the *fight-or-flight response*. It is a mixed blessing. Without it, we would not be able to counter danger, take advantage of opportunities, or feel excitement. Indeed, we might not survive at all without the stress response. However, the same response, especially if prolonged or repeated often, may lead to physical symptoms, including headache. A person who sees many things—perhaps almost everything—as a challenge or threat will experience excessive and potentially harmful stress.

Emotional arousal is one of the most common triggers for migraine and tension-type headache. For the headache sufferer it is not necessary that this stress be excessive, although if it is the risk seems to rise accordingly. If you are prone to headache, even normal levels of stress can set off a headache attack. Positive as well as negative arousal can be a trigger for a migraine headache. The trigger may operate by way of underlying activity in the brain itself or by the effects of tension on other parts of the body such as the muscles, which become tense, leading to pain. Prolonged tension may lead to depression, which makes the whole system more vulnerable to headaches.

You may already know whether you tend to build up excessive internal tension. If you find that you often can answer yes to the following questions (and you are otherwise in good health), you may have higher headache risk due to chronically high internal tension. If so, it may be important to consider the sources of this chronic tension—in your environment and/or in your way of living in your world—and make some changes. Whether or not you are a chronically tense person, you can use this list to evaluate tension level at any particular time. Affirmative answers should tell you it's time to relax, to interrupt the building tension.

Is My Body Sending Me Stress Warning Signals?

+ Does my heartbeat feel fast or pounding?
+ Is it hard for me to catch my breath or take a full breath?
+ Do I find myself holding my breath?
+ Am I breathing faster than I need to?
+ Is my energy level unusually high or low?
+ Did I wake up tired?
+ Did I have trouble getting to sleep? Did I wake up too early?
+ Can I feel my face flushing?

+ Does my neck feel tight, stiff, or sore?
+ Are my shoulders tense, raised, or pulled forward?
+ Am I clenching my teeth? Frowning?
+ Are my fingers colder than usual? (Press them against your cheeks. How cold do they feel?)
+ Am I having trouble concentrating?
+ Is my mind too busy thinking of what I don't have time for? Am I feeling overwhelmed?
+ Am I going from one task to another aimlessly?
+ Am I worrying about what is not done right? About what I have done myself or what others have done?
+ Am I unable to stop thinking about unfair situations or unspoken conflicts?
+ Am I talking faster than usual?
+ Am I eating too much? Or do I just have no appetite at all?
+ Are others asking me to calm down or slow down?
+ Do I feel irritable? Anxious? Angry? Very excited? Fearful? Guilty? Drained? Embarrassed? Filled with dread? Sad?
+ Is the emotion understandable given the current situation? Is this the kind of emotion I feel often?
+ Am I feeling stronger emotion than necessary for the immediate situation?

Relaxation serves many purposes. In its extended form it is a way of letting go of tension and feeling deep calm and peacefulness. You might think of this form of relaxation as a deep well to which you come to fill your canteen. In the course of daily life, relaxation must be done more briefly. In this form you are breaking the building tension. You might think of it as taking a sip from that canteen as you move along your path. Both forms of relaxation are important. In the first you build your skills and restore your body and mind. In the second you catch tension before it becomes too great, letting go of it when the crisis is past or keeping arousal to the least necessary level appropriate to the situation.

WHAT RELAXATION IS—AND ISN'T

Some people reject the idea of relaxation as a treatment, thinking we are suggesting they just be calm when the pain of a headache strikes. This, of course, is not the idea at all. It does help to stay as relaxed as possible while working with medication and other techniques to control a headache that has already started. But the most important application of relaxation is in preventing headaches in the first place or catching signs of a headache early so that you can head it off.

Others protest that they have no time for relaxation, believing that we are just advocating more time off—at the golf course or the beach. Understandably this won't seem practical to all those with work and family obligations. While adequate recreation is important to leading a balanced life, taking time away from responsibilities is not what we mean by relaxation. Relaxation, as we use the term, is a way of doing whatever you are engaged in, and you'll find your relaxation training useful in approaching all the tasks of your daily life, including work, taking care of family, and negotiating weekly shopping forays.

For still others, relaxation is mistakenly equated with simply "vegging out." Putting up your feet, having a cool drink, and watching your favorite television show may not be a bad diversion, but it is not what we mean by relaxation training. In the therapeutic sense relaxation means the reduction of the physical, mental, emotional, and behavioral aspects of unnecessary arousal. In fact relaxation training is sometimes called *low-arousal training.* When you successfully achieve deep relaxation, many changes can be measured or reported. Your hands and feet become warmer, muscles relax, breathing and heart rate slow, blood pressure drops, thinking becomes more tranquil, emotions more manageable. There are many subtle changes in body chemistry as well, all leading to reduction of the stress response and to reduction of risk for headache.

Some of us are born with bodies that become tense more easily or don't let go of tension. Our physical tendency is aggravated or ameliorated by the way we have learned to think about ourselves and our world. You may be a person who relaxes easily and often each day, responding only to the demands of the immediate situation. You may be able to let go of anger or fear as soon as the danger or challenge is past. On the other hand you may react quickly and strongly, finding it very difficult to relax even when you have "won." However you find yourself today, all of us can develop a greater capacity to relax. With competent training and diligent practice the relaxation response can become an almost automatic reaction to the stresses of your life. In this way you develop great facility at preventing some headaches, catching others early and thus allowing for behavioral and medical intervention before pain becomes severe, or at least limiting the suffering involved in severe headaches that do break through.

METHODS OF RELAXATION

In the course of your initial evaluations at a comprehensive headache clinic, your overall psychological and social situation will be considered. Typically the psychologist will review the recurring stressors you recognize in your life, your usual coping methods, and the intensity and types of stress responses you usually have. Most people already try to relax when internal tension is high, and how successful you are in this effort is also important information. Based on this review, the psychologist will establish a practical treatment plan. This plan will have several levels of intervention. You will be asked to include some rating of your stress or relaxation level in your headache diary. This allows you to better recognize the stress response, determine the typical stress level, and begin to see with what internal or external events the stress reactions are associated. As you recognize recurring events, you will develop cognitive-behavioral strategies to change them or your way of handling them. This will be discussed in more detail in Chapter 9. In this chapter, we will be discussing the other key element of the plan, learning the relaxation response itself.

The psychological or behavioral treatment plan is most often carried out by the psychologist or by the biobehavioral therapist under the supervision of the psychologist. In training the relaxation response the therapist will try to build the skills systematically. The first task is extended training in relaxation. For this purpose the therapist will spend time in the office taking you through the entire relaxation exercise. A taped set of instructions is often introduced, which you can then use at home as well. Because relaxation is first a skill that is learned, practice at home is essential. Office practice is not sufficient; your life will not change because you spend one hour a week feeling relaxed. In the office, biofeedback equipment is often used to ensure that the relaxation not only feels good but has an effect on the bodily signs of arousal or relaxation as well. Biofeedback will be discussed later in this chapter. As you develop a reliable relaxation response in the extended practice, you will be trained to relax more on your own, without the tape or biofeedback. Gradually you'll learn a brief relaxation response that can be used practically in the course of your daily life.

As you learn to relax more often and more effectively, and as you maintain your headache diary with the stress levels noted, gradually and almost imperceptibly you'll develop a new awareness. You'll become better able to recognize accurately smaller and smaller changes in your level of internal tension. This ability to be in touch with your body, which we call *accurate somatic awareness*, is of great benefit to people with headaches. You will find yourself able to catch tension early, even before it becomes transformed into the pain of headache. By catching tension early and responding effectively, you prevent or cut off a greater proportion of your headaches, especially those triggered by the stress response.

As we've noted, there are many forms of relaxation. The one you use should be the one that feels most comfortable to you and still gets results where it counts, in the reduction of physical and mental stress and the reduction in frequency and severity of headache. We will describe here some of the more common methods of relaxation. These are tried-and-true methods that have worked for many people. The description in this chapter will be brief, just enough to give you the flavor. If you find a method that seems compatible with you, learn more about it by pursuing some of the references listed at the end of this book.

If you do seek treatment in a comprehensive headache clinic, or with a psychologist otherwise familiar with headaches, he or she will introduce you to a variety of written and taped materials that will help you select and learn a combination of relaxation techniques right for you. In our own clinic we often begin with a very reliable technique called *progressive muscle relaxation* but add or substitute other techniques as the patient requires or wishes. The end is more important than the route by which you reach it.

Whichever form of relaxation you set out to learn, two elements seem to be important in mastering the basic technique. First, the environment in which you practice must encourage relaxation. Find a chair that supports your body without putting you to sleep. To really let go of your conscious attention to detail and focus on your body, you will need relative quiet and freedom from interruption. The temperature and lighting should be comfortable. You may have to make arrangements with other family members to have this time to yourself. And there is a reason the telephone has a jack. Television or talk radio is not a suitable background for learning relaxation, but soothing music will do nicely. New Age tapes or music from the classical/baroque period usually promotes relaxation optimally.

Second, you must learn to adopt an attitude of consciously setting out to relax but not trying too hard. This somewhat paradoxical combination of intention and passivity has been called *passive volition*. *Volition* implies that you intend to relax; that is the reason you have come to this point. *Passive* recognizes that you cannot force relaxation; you can only become quiet enough to let it happen. For a physical example, consider muscle relaxation; you don't relax muscles as much as you stop tensing them. The relaxation then follows on its own. Remember this as you learn the details of each method, then try to put them into practice. A method of relaxation is not a sequence of mechanical steps that directly produces relaxation. Rather, it is a set of guidelines to help you experience this elusive idea of letting go. Biofeedback should be viewed this way too: it is more useful as a source of accurate information about how you are doing in relaxing than as a new task by which to achieve relaxation.

One word of caution: Unexpectedly, relaxation exercises have been found to produce a state of anxiety in some individuals. Usually there are identifiable reasons for this anxiety. Old and unwanted memories may surface. Being so unguarded may feel very uncomfortable. Taking time for yourself or being "unproductive" may give rise to guilt. If you find yourself anxious as you practice the relaxation techniques described in this book, stop and take the experience to a psychologist or counselor familiar with relaxation to process your reactions. Finding and working through the reasons for your anxiety requires professional assistance.

Physical Methods

The following two methods—progressive muscle relaxation and deep breathing—focus on physical events as paths to relaxation. These two methods are very reliable. They have been useful for a wide range of people, and many therapists start with them to introduce the idea of relaxation. Some people find all they need in these basic methods, while others go on to further physical or mental techniques as well.

Progressive Relaxation

In addition to being described in almost any book on relaxation methods, progressive relaxation is the focus of many audiotapes. When developed by Edmund Jacobson in 1938, the technique was described as detailed and lengthy, but it is now typically taught in more abbreviated versions. Muscle groups are combined in various ways, and mental suggestion is used to enhance general relaxation of the nervous system.

Progressive relaxation involves purposefully tensing and then relaxing groups of muscles in a definite sequence, or progression. From a comfortable lying or sitting position, for example, you might begin with the right fist, clenching the fist tightly for three to five seconds, then slowly releasing the fist and feeling the sensations of relaxation as you do so. Try it yourself and see how it feels. You would then do the same with the left fist, letting the right hand remain relaxed. Progressing through all the muscle groups of your body, you maintain your awareness of the sensations of tension and relaxation, encouraging with your attention (no effort!) the building sense of relaxation that gradually spreads to all areas of your body.

The entire sequence in the forms most commonly practiced today will take about twenty to thirty minutes. You are asked to practice the technique once or twice each day as you learn it. Abbreviated forms are available once you thoroughly master the basic technique. As reliable and common as progressive muscle relaxation is, it is still not for everyone. The muscles of some people are so stiff and tender that purposefully tensing them actually increases pain. If you fall into this group, you will have to use other methods until physical therapy can make enough headway that the muscles are not so vulnerable to irritation.

Deep Breathing

Breathing is so basic that we think about it only when it becomes difficult. The idea that you could benefit from training in breathing may seem strange, yet this basic act, essential to life itself, is often done less than optimally. Perhaps for many people the less efficient breathing pattern is not critical, but for the person with chronic tension or the headache sufferer who wishes to keep internal tension to a minimum, more efficient breathing is a useful tool for relaxation.

When we speak of deep breathing we mean neither taking great gulps of air nor magnificently expanding the chest as you might see on a cartoon. *Deep* actually refers to breathing from the bottom of your lungs up. The area at the base of the lungs is the most efficient at transferring oxygen to the bloodstream. In addition, deep breathing implies effortless breathing, just the opposite of exaggerated gulping of air. While you might intermittently take an exaggerated breath to break tension, the rhythm of deep breathing is actually very slow, about ten breaths per minute or so, longer on the exhale than the inhale, and with hardly observable movement except for the abdomen going in and out. We will describe some aspects of the technique, but remember that more important than any specific rule is the idea of breathing effortlessly, gracefully.

This can literally be done anywhere and anytime except when you must exert yourself forcefully.

To help you relax through deep breathing, your therapist will help you focus first on the alternation of tension and relaxation. As you breathe in, you will feel the tension of the abdominal and chest walls. As you breathe out, letting go rather than forcefully expelling air, you will feel the movement to relaxation. Just let the air slowly seep out, like a slow leak from a tire. Move gradually to a slower and slower pace of breathing. You will find you don't need so much oxygen as you relax physically, mentally, and emotionally. If at times you feel tense or starved for air, break the tension by taking one of those large and visible breaths, let the air out slowly, and start again. If you can, breathe in through your nose and out through gently pursed lips.

As mentioned, your goal is seeking to take air all the way to the bottom of your lungs. To do this, it is most efficient to breathe by flattening the diaphragm, the muscular lining between the lung cavity and the abdominal cavity. As you do so, you will see the abdominal wall expand. With fuller breaths, the rib cage will naturally expand as well. This method of diaphragmatic breathing may also be called *stomach* or *belly breathing*. This does not mean, of course, that you are breathing with your stomach. It just refers to the fact that when you breathe by expanding or flattening the diaphragm your abdominal wall protrudes slightly.

An Exercise to Test Your Breathing Pattern. In the beginning, it may seem awkward or uncomfortable to breathe in this way. You may feel you cannot do it. Remember again that no particular style of breathing is more important than your sense of ease—just focus first on breathing slowly, in through your nose if possible and out through your slightly pursed lips. Then move toward more and more effortless breathing, finding a rhythm and method that feel right to you. Your therapist can help you evaluate the successfulness of your pattern using biofeedback equipment, described later in this chapter.

To learn how to breathe with your diaphragm, consider an old technique taught by meditation masters. Lie down on your back, with one hand on your chest and the other on your abdomen. Sip in air with your mouth, as if you were using a straw. Focus on the movement of your lower hand compared with the upper hand. Notice especially when the lower hand moves up with inhalation and down with exhalation while the upper hand remains relatively still. When the upper hand moves more than the lower, just exhale and focus on the next time. In this way you will gradually reinforce successful diaphragmatic breathing.

Nonrelaxing Breathing Patterns. Your therapist may also caution you against some unhelpful ways of breathing. One of these is hyperventilation, which results from forced breathing—breathing that is too deep and/or rapid. Hyperventilation can be very obvious—a person who is very frightened, for example, may breathe so rapidly that the noise and effort are unmistakable. More often, hyperventilation is subtle, resulting from poor breathing habits. Sometimes people learning to deep-breathe will misunderstand and breathe deeply at a normal rate. Hyperventilation leads to excessive amounts of oxygen relative to carbon dioxide in your bloodstream. It is associated with high arousal, the opposite of the state you seek with relaxation. In this state it is not unusual to experience symptoms of anxiety, light-headedness, and even panic.

We call breathing by expanding and/or raising the chest wall *thoracic (chest)* or *clavicular breathing.* In this very common pattern of breathing the diaphragm's role in inhalation is reduced. Lung capacity is not used as efficiently. Sometimes people think this type of breathing is more natural or looks better. Many of us learn to worry about our stomach protruding under any circumstances! Don't worry; your stomach will not get any larger from diaphragmatic breathing, and it is far more efficient than chest breathing.

Engaging the Mind and Body

The next group of methods uses cognitive or mental techniques as well as physical methods to encourage relaxation. You may find that these methods do not come as naturally as did progressive relaxation or deep breathing. They rely more on your unique personal history and your ability to manipulate mental images. Some of you may take to them very easily, while others may require considerable coaching to allow images to form or phrases to resonate in your mind. If you find that you have difficulty with these methods but want to explore them further, we encourage you to seek guidance from a therapist trained in their use. The rewards can be rich for the person who masters the art of nonverbal expression.

On the other hand, don't feel pressured to learn them. There is no point in forcing yourself to relax in any way. Again, the end is more important than the particular method you select. In a comprehensive headache clinic it is your therapist's job to help you find the method or methods that will work for you. Just speak up if you don't like a method, even if it is introduced with great enthusiasm.

Imagery

Imagery is hard to define. It has been described simply as pictures formed in the mind, or the sensory imagination. Since imagery typically requires some idea of what relaxation feels like, many therapists use it as a follow-up to progressive relaxation and/or deep breathing. Your therapist may first suggest progressive relaxation and/or deep breathing and then ask you to deepen that relaxation through the use of imagery. Imagery can be used in many ways to promote relaxation.

Focused Imagery. This method involves focusing on a part of the body that is particularly tense. You might begin by scanning your body slowly, from head to toes, with your "mind's eye" (your eyes closed). Focus first on the relaxed parts of the body and enjoy them. Then turn to the tense parts, one at a time. Imagine relaxing events occurring in that part. For example, if your neck muscles are tight, your therapist might suggest that you feel them being worked by an unseen hand or many small creatures all at your command. If your head feels as though it is surrounded by a tight band, imagine it slowly being loosened. You can be as fanciful as you care to be, but imagine the events in detail and feel them actually taking place at each step. If your hands are cold, imagine a warming beach sun baking them as you lie calmly. Hear the surf in the background and feel the sleepiness taking over your body. You get the idea. Try it out. Your therapist can monitor your activity with biofeedback equipment to be sure that you are in fact learning an effective technique; you should just enjoy it.

Deepening Imagery. In this method your focus is on the body as a whole rather than on separate parts. Imagine a large thermometer, with the lowest level representing a high level of tension and the highest a deep relaxation. As you scan your body, find your level of relaxation along the thermometer. Then as you relax, allow your current level to rise. Wherever you start, imagine what it would feel like to reach the next notch and let yourself start to feel it so. Just keep going up, little by little. Let it happen; don't force it. Feel it happening; don't try to think your way to relaxation.

Guided Imagery. With this method you create and experience in your mind a place that you feel would be spontaneously relaxing—a supportive environment. With the help of your therapist, you might choose a place of beauty, tranquillity, and security, a place where soothing sensations are near, anxiety and tension far away. It might be a placid mountain lake in which great mountains, blue sky, yellow sun, and slowly passing white clouds are reflected. It might be any place that is relaxing to you, real or fantasized. Once you are there, your therapist may ask you to focus on each of your senses—to see, hear, touch, smell, and taste so fully that you experience the place more deeply. Relaxation simply follows the heightened sensation; let it flow through all parts of your body and mind.

Role-Playing Imagery. This method is often reserved for a later phase in relaxation training, once you have acquired some skill at relaxing through other methods. Again you are asked to visualize a place, but this time a place where you have encountered stress in your life. Once you have the place and situation in mind, your therapist may ask you to imagine responding to the situation in a more relaxed way—in other words, to play a different and more beneficial role. For example, imagine yourself in your office with a difficult co-worker. You are supportive but firm with this person and feel confident and relaxed about the outcome of your meeting.

Role-playing imagery allows you to rehearse mentally how you would like to behave in stressful circumstances and to learn what it feels like to be more relaxed in those situations. This makes it ideal for generalization, a phase of relaxation training discussed later in this chapter in which you take relaxation from your training and practice site to all the places in which you normally encounter stress. With role-playing imagery you can generalize to other settings mentally before going on to try it out literally.

Alternative Methods

The following techniques are powerful but may be more difficult to learn for the inexperienced relaxer trying them alone. A biobehavioral therapist or other guide may be particularly useful in understanding and working through obstacles to progress. As with all the relaxation exercises, if you experience sensations that are uncomfortable or produce anxiety, just stop. Ask your therapist for help.

Meditation

Meditation is an old and honored discipline that can be learned in a multitude of forms, many of which can be used to promote relaxation. When it is taught in a biobehavioral therapist's office for the purpose of headache management, it is often taught in an abbreviated form with an emphasis on clearing your mind, letting go of stressful thoughts and images.

To meditate effectively you need a supportive environment and a comfortable sitting or lying position, as you do with all the methods described here. A receptive mental attitude will serve you, going beyond the concept of passive volition described earlier. Here you abandon even the desire to make anything in particular happen in your mind. When thoughts and images enter your awareness, you are asked simply to let them go by without focusing on them. You also remain unconcerned about how well you are doing at meditation. Success is simply a state of mental being, not an achievement.

If you have heard a little about transcendental meditation, you're familiar with the concept of a mantra, a word or sound repeated periodically during meditation. A mantra is only one possible choice; any object that you can focus on will do. A mantra is used because the sound object is brief (one syllable), is easily repeatable, and has no strong meaning or association in itself. It serves mainly to focus your attention away from any stressful thoughts and images that may enter your mind during meditation. With a visual object you fix your gaze on it to clear your awareness of extraneous matters.

Both meditation and imagery are based on the idea that ridding the mind of stressful thoughts can help the body let go of its stress response and allow the relaxation response to emerge. The two methods simply go about this in different ways. Imagery tries to replace thoughts of stress or tension with more relaxing images. Meditation tries to induce a state of quiet and clarity in which the mind no longer holds on to stressful thoughts and images but rather allows them to drift away. With either technique the desired outcome is a mental state conducive to relaxation.

Autogenic Training

This method consists of a series of phrases intended to focus your attention on the relaxed sensations of your body. Like progressive relaxation, it was introduced as an extensive and systematic method of relaxing the body and promoting health. However, autogenic training is now usually taught in a much more abbreviated form. Here it is presented in a sample series of six phrases. During a given relaxation period you would be asked to hear one or more of these phrases repeated in your mind.

1. My arms and legs are heavy.
2. My arms and legs are warm.
3. My heartbeat is calm and regular.
4. It breathes me.
5. My abdomen is warm.
6. My forehead is cool.

As with progressive relaxation, your therapist may have you begin with just one of these phrases, moving on to the next one after you are able to hear the phrase and feel the physical change. There are many different ways of organizing the basic phrases. How you say or "hear" the phrases in your mind is important. Rote recitation will accomplish little. The experience is more aptly described as hearing the phrases being said in your mind, and you must allow yourself to feel the sensations described. Phrase 4, "It breathes me," might be difficult to understand. However, it is a powerful phrase in which the sensation is one of your breathing becoming so effortless and natural that it may seem as though someone or something else is doing the breathing. After your initial period of training, you may be able to go through an effective sequence of autogenic phrases in as little as ten minutes. In sessions where you have more time, your therapist may encourage you to deepen the result of the autogenic sequence, feeling your body almost asleep while your mind is awake.

Brief Relaxation

Brief relaxation is not a method in itself but a way of transforming any method to make it more useful in everyday life. As mentioned, it is not enough to be able to relax effectively in your therapist's office or even at your home practice site. You must be able to use relaxation when you notice early signs of tension, to move you away from building tension and toward relaxation. It doesn't matter that the depth of relaxation is not great at that moment. What is important is that you are stopping the upward spiral of tension. You will learn to use brief relaxation frequently and unobtrusively. It doesn't matter how often you must do so; just don't give in to the tension you feel.

Early in treatment your therapist is likely to introduce one- to five-minute techniques for you to use. Of course, you will be able to employ them more effectively as you get a better idea of the sensations of relaxation and are more able to recognize their opposite, the early signs of tension. Brief relaxation is often taught as a brief "ritual" with discrete parts. It commonly begins with a scan of your body to identify areas of tension, poor posture, or ineffective breathing. Next you may slow your breathing rate and allow yourself to exhale slowly and imperceptibly. Then you might visualize specific areas of tension relaxing as you exhale and/or adjust your posture. As you can see, brief relaxation is often a composite of the more extensive relaxation methods you will have learned.

Once you and your therapist have come up with a brief relaxation procedure that you can use without special equipment or guidance wherever you may be, you will be encouraged to begin practicing it at home and at work—wherever and whenever you perceive the early signs of tension. You may be asked to use the procedure simply to enhance relaxation, whether you feel tension or not, practicing a one-minute brief relaxation as often as fifty to a hundred times a day. The repetition of these brief exercises reinforces the training you receive in your therapist's office, makes you more aware of sources of stress and tension in your daily life, and helps you incorporate relaxation into your lifestyle so you can reduce your risk of headache.

As with the other modes of therapy discussed in this book, relaxation is most effective when you actively collaborate with your therapist. Relaxation is not something that is done *to* you; it is a skill for you to learn and a tool for you to use. Depend on your biobehavioral therapist's knowledge of various techniques and of the most effective ways to learn relaxation, but realize that it is up to you to develop the habits that allow you to practice the techniques at home and use them in the course of everyday life. You may use a variety of methods over time, changing as you advance in skill or develop preferences. Usually, as your training continues, you will form a routine or a sequence of methods to use when you want to practice relaxation for an extended period or employ brief relaxation.

Relaxation is not a quick fix; it requires a long-term commitment. If you find that you don't take so easily to relaxation as a discipline, the good news is that you need not continue to practice it as extensively later in treatment. Once your headaches are under some control, you must only maintain an awareness of tension and keep up the habit of brief relaxation.

BIOFEEDBACK AND RELAXATION

How will you and your therapist know when a method of relaxation is working for you? How can you be sure a relaxation exercise or routine leaves you with lowered arousal? Commonsense observations such as a more relaxed feeling, lessening of pain, and decreasing frequency or intensity of headache may be signs. You will also learn more subtle cues, like warming hands or a general sense of heaviness. But your sense that you are relaxing is not always reliable. It is possible to feel you are relaxing when your body is in fact still quite tense. Biofeedback provides an excellent tool for learning and assessing the quality of relaxation. It is an invaluable tool in any biobehavioral therapy—behavioral treatment to affect physical activity.

Biofeedback means literally the provision (or feeding back to you) of information about your body's (biological) current state. This information may be provided in any number of ways, both natural and artificial. When we speak of biofeedback, we typically refer to methods created by human beings for measuring physical events that are not easy to assess through our natural sensory processes. Today we're also usually referring to the use of sensitive electronic instruments that measure even small changes in the body and provide the information very quickly (in real time).

Biofeedback is a very important and useful tool in teaching relaxation or low arousal. In this case the instruments are selected to provide information about how successfully you are relaxing muscles or reducing sympathetic nervous system activity. You then use the information to enhance your ability to experience relaxation. We believe this way of thinking about biofeedback is much more effective and realistic than ideas that biofeedback is a relaxation method in itself. Biofeedback clearly does not do anything to you. It is not like receiving a massage or taking a pill. It is a teaching tool that provides information to therapist and patient about the success of the relaxation methods employed. The information can be reinforcing when given to you in ways that promote learning—that is, the machines can encourage you in realizing the control you do have over your body and the extent to which you can learn to be sensitive to the messages of your body. There are also some general effects of being hooked up to scientific machines that may actually make you more confident in the relaxation procedure and thus increase its effects. But in the end biofeedback is best seen as a tool, augmenting your relaxation training, rather than as a new procedure.

Biofeedback instruments provide their information to you in many ways. The more common forms of the feedback are visual or auditory— you may be given a meter or bar to view, for example, or be asked to listen to a sound that rises or falls in pitch. Biofeedback may also be used to measure many different kinds of physical events. In the following paragraphs we will give you a general picture of four kinds of instruments that you are most likely to encounter while learning relaxation for headache management. The particular instruments your therapist will use with you will depend on many factors, including the physical responses that are most pronounced in you. He or she may begin with a brief assessment to determine which physical measures are likely to be most revealing in your particular case.

Thermograph

One of the general effects of reduced arousal is increased blood flow to the fingers and toes. This results from relaxation of the smooth muscle around the small blood vessels in these areas; the vessels then increase in size as the blood is pumped into the area. More blood results in warmer temperatures at the surface. As a result of these processes, measurement of skin temperature at the fingertips is one reliable and simple measure of the effectiveness of relaxation. Of course, this assumes that the room temperature is steady and not at either extreme and that you have no medical condition that otherwise impairs blood flow to the fingers.

Electromyograph

This measure, usually called *EMG*, reflects the amount of electrical activity produced by your muscles. As muscles tense, they produce electrical activity that can be measured at the surface of your skin. Therefore, the less electrical activity measured, the more relaxed the muscle at that moment. The sensors are taped over a particular muscle group. How they are placed makes a big difference in how much activity will be detected and how it can be interpreted. The machine itself also has a number of settings that affect the amount of electrical activity that can be measured.

Electrodermograph

This measurement is based on the increase in sweat gland activity at the hands that typically occurs when we are aroused or tense. This measurement can be accomplished in several ways. One is based on the electrical activity itself; others are based on the amount of moisture on the skin. This measure tends to be highly variable from moment to moment during a relaxation session. It may be used in conjunction with the skin temperature measurement. The idea is to learn to keep your hands warm and dry.

Electroencephalograph

This tongue twister is commonly called an *EEG*. Physicians use it for diagnostic purposes. In biobehavioral therapy the EEG is used to measure the dominant frequency of brain electrical activity. Sensors are placed on your scalp to measure the activity. In general, low or high arousal can be associated with different dominant frequencies of brain electrical activity. The goal is low-frequency electrical activity during relaxation practice.

✦

Biofeedback instruments from well-known companies and used by trained technicians are quite safe. Much effort has gone into the design of such equipment to make them usable in many settings outside special laboratories or medical buildings. Although many of the measures are based on electrical activity, there is protection against the introduction of harmful levels of electricity into your body. For the most part, biofeedback instruments measure naturally occurring electrical activity from your own body and convert it into information that you can see and use.

For their purpose, biofeedback instruments are exceptionally useful. They provide information to therapist and patient that keeps both on the course toward effective relaxation skills and accurate physical awareness. These two abilities are essential building blocks for the behavioral part of headache management. On the other hand, it is equally important not to give the machines more credit than they deserve. Even when the treatment is called biofeedback, the machines themselves are not the treatment. As you learn an effective relaxation regimen and are able to recognize levels of tension more accurately and sensitively, the equipment will be withdrawn gradually. You will move to independence from the biofeedback. First the feedback may be turned off, moving to the oral guidance of the therapist only. Then you will learn to relax independently, checking in only intermittently to see how you are doing. The overall movement is always toward internalization of the relaxation process and increased sensitivity to signs of tension. It is important that you be able to relax in many settings, not just in your therapist's office, and that you be able to interrupt building tension even when you cannot take the time for a full period of relaxation. We hope these basic skills lead then to a more relaxed approach to life in general. As you recognize and work with the early signs of tension, you will naturally awake to the recurring sources of tension in your life, internal or external. To put it in the vocabulary of our profession, we want you to generalize your relaxation training.

GENERALIZING YOUR RELAXATION TRAINING

Chronic headache, even when treated successfully, cannot be cured. Effective treatment implies lifelong changes in the way you think of your headache syndrome, the way you relate to your body, what you expect from your physician and other health professionals, and how you view your role in the treatment or management of your headache. One of these changes is the generalization of relaxation.

Generalizing relaxation training has many dimensions. We have been talking about learning to relax without the biofeedback and outside of the therapist's office. We noted our desire that you should learn to relax even apart from extended relaxation sessions, taking the calmness you have learned there to many parts of your day. Sometimes the ultimate goal has been described as learning an *attitude* of relaxation, incorporating relaxation into your way of living.

There are many behavioral supports to this process of generalization. An early assignment is to establish daily practice sessions. Carving out this time ensures that at least at that point in your day you will remove yourself from the flow of daily stressors, finding some comfort and privacy other than in the therapist's office. Soon thereafter you may be asked to use a system by which you are reminded frequently to stop for a moment to check your body, thoughts, and feelings for signs of tension and to use a brief relaxation ritual. These brief sessions—some as short as one minute—may occur many times each day. They may be triggered by any familiar stress-augmenting activity of your day. For example, brief relaxation may be called for each time you look at your watch or whenever the phone rings.

Your ongoing process of recordkeeping is also a great aid to generalization. As you record not only pain but your activities, eating pattern, feelings, and sensations of physical tension, you will also become more sensitive to yourself. The pattern that emerges will help you identify early signs of tension and even anticipate tension at certain times or in particular places or situations. With each step you come closer to the ultimate goal of generalization—the incorporation of relaxation into your lifestyle.

As you do so, your therapist will help you modify the recurring sources of tension. Perhaps you need new skills. For example, recurring stress at work may call for increased assertiveness. Overwork may signal the need for improved social skills or increased self-esteem. It may be that you must unlearn certain thought patterns or reflexive behaviors. For example, you may have a pattern of interpreting the comments of others as critical or demeaning, leading to seething resentment. You may need to unlearn a habit of responding to every perceived need of others, learning to assess first what they really need or want. Perhaps you must change the pace at which you habitually approach your day. Can you learn to vary your pace to accommodate different conditions inside your body or in your environment? These are just a few examples of more extensive changes in the way you live, rising from the basic relaxation training and recordkeeping, that will help you truly generalize relaxation and self-care. Taking control of your headaches moves from just managing symptoms to really *living* with your headache syndrome. The actual relaxation practice will change over time, and as you get your headaches under better control, you will not need to practice as extensively if you don't wish to. These basic changes in behavior and thinking, however, will be part of you for the rest of your life. Our discussion of the behavioral therapies in Chapter 9 will give you a more extensive picture of this level of generalization.

✦ THE CASE OF KAREN L., PART 5

You may recall that Karen L. told her doctors at her initial evaluation that she felt "stuck" trying to work, go to school, and raise three children all at the same time. Her doctors described this feeling to her as internal tension, aggravating the headache syndrome directly and by way of the increased muscle tension it caused. So, as she began a course in physical therapy (described in Chapter 7), she also entered biobehavioral therapy, which included relaxation training.

Her doctors believed the two modalities would work together to reduce Karen's muscle tension and internal tension—and thus help her take control of her headaches.

Karen's progress proved them right. After initial therapy sessions in which her pattern of arousal was assessed with biofeedback equipment, she was taught progressive relaxation and autogenic relaxation. She was given audiotapes to help her in home practice and asked to work with them for at least half an hour a day. In their sessions together, Karen's therapist used the electromyograph (EMG), with the sensors placed in the area between the base of her neck and her shoulder joint on both sides of her body, to measure Karen's habitual use of the muscles in that area. The EMG indicated that Karen unknowingly overused the muscles on the left side, even when she was trying to relax. Letting the muscle relax even hurt somewhat since it was not used to being stretched. This was helpful information to her physical therapist, and it provided some of the focus for the relaxation training as well. The biofeedback instrument, combined with some old-fashioned visual feedback of sitting in front of a mirror while practicing, helped her recognize the internal cues of muscle tension in this area. With encouragement she used this awareness with the stretching exercises from her physical therapist to carry her shoulder in a way that allowed for appropriate reduction of muscle tension. At first this ability was limited mostly to the therapist's office. At school and work, Karen reported, she had some difficulty remembering and being able to accomplish the same thing. She wondered if she would ever be able to relax with so many distractions.

Skin temperature feedback while relaxing indicated that she was learning the basic skill. Her therapist then proceeded to increase her competence and confidence in relaxing by gradually removing the feedback and oral encouragement while she relaxed. In their sessions, with help from her therapist, she learned also to identify muscle tension at the left shoulder without the biofeedback. At home she began to find that her relaxation exercises were more effective and took some well-deserved satisfaction from regularly giving herself this break from her day. In the course of her workday she began at least to recognize early signs of a headache and even of tension, responding to them with medicine when appropriate but always by relaxing her body and taking stock of the sources of the current tension, internal or external.

By the end of the first month, as Chapter 7 stated, Karen's headaches had improved dramatically. Karen's practice of progressive and autogenic relaxation, reinforced by skin temperature biofeedback, had resulted in lower overall internal tension, reducing her risk of headache. Her EMG biofeedback, focusing on the left shoulder, had complemented her physical therapy and lowered her muscle tension in that area. The muscles were irritated less easily, further reducing her risk factors for headache. The use of brief relaxation and frequent checks of her level of tension had started to help her generalize the basic relaxation. She was interrupting building tension and learning the recurring sources of tension in her life. As just one example, in school she noticed that her left shoulder tension increased when her attention was focused on a difficult concept. Her body position habitually shifted so that her head was leaning to the left side and the shoulder rose to meet it. Even her jaw was set and shifted to the left as she concentrated. Part of her practice in generalizing, whenever she recognized this pattern, was to stop, assume a more relaxed posture, breathe deeply and slowly, then return to concentrating only with her mind, leaving her body in a more relaxed state. "Focused but not tense" was the phrase she used to help herself regroup.

In the next chapter we will address one remaining dimension of Karen's generalization of relaxation: changing ways of coping with recurrent psychosocial or other stressors that lead to increased arousal and thereby trigger or increase the overall risk of headaches.

✦

CHAPTER 9

Minimize Psychosocial Stress: Cognitive-Behavioral Therapy

WhEN we left Karen L. in Chapter 8, she was successfully generalizing her relaxation training. That is, she was beginning to take the techniques she had learned in her therapist's office to many parts of her life—home, work, and school. As we've seen, relaxation training, physical therapy, and medication changes had been used in an integrated way (multimodal treatment) to decrease the frequency of Karen's headaches considerably. Both Karen and her treatment team were gratified by the results of their coordinated efforts. Yet all agreed that the process of treatment was not complete. Further progress could be made, with greater assurance that the effect of treatment would endure.

The next phase of treatment, as we suggested at the end of Chapter 8, lay in the extension of Karen's biobehavioral therapy, using the methods of cognitive-behavioral therapy to address the recurring stressors triggering or generally increasing her risk of headaches. In some way, of course, all the modes of therapy we have covered so far—medication, physical therapy, and relaxation training—have cognitive and behavioral elements. Each involves a conceptual understanding of headache and requires that you think about how to use it. Each has a behavioral element, requiring that you actually perform the prescribed acts, whether that is taking a particular medicine, performing an exercise, or taking the time for relaxation. When we speak of cognitive-behavioral therapy in this chapter, however, we mean an extension of the biobehavioral therapy that began with relaxation and recordkeeping and progressed through more accurate and timely awareness of your bodily reactions to the application of relaxation in everyday life.

Many gains occur, as they did for Karen L., just from these first phases of biobehavioral therapy. Generalization of relaxation is like a flood of water rushing through a dry creek bed. Much silt and other loose material is washed away. However, you also come up against the hard places, the rocks in the creek bed. These are the recurring sources of stress in your life. They may be particularly virulent stressors or other triggers of headaches. They may be situations calling for skills that are just not your strengths. They may touch parts of your personal history that are particularly painful for you and have not been worked through. There may be competing needs or goals that leave you in conflict.

In such situations, simply continuing to use relaxation alone will probably not be efficient. Certainly relaxation could help, but it would not be getting to the root of the problem. Consider a home in winter that has become unbearably hot. Opening the windows, as helpful as that may be in the short run, would be a very inefficient long-term solution, analogous to using only the relaxation portion of biobehavioral therapy. The role of cognitive-behavioral therapy, in contrast, is to identify and resolve the sources of recurrent stress—akin to finding the thermostat and turning it down. Your difficulties may lie largely in the situation itself or may originate in your own past. The changes you will need to make may be in your way of thinking about the situation, your way of responding to it, or the emotions you experience. You may be called on to modify or learn a particular behavior or to adjust an entire style of being or relating in the world. Cognitive-behavioral therapy is not the only way to address such problems, but it is a particularly good fit as a component of biobehavioral therapy and is perhaps the most commonly used approach in comprehensive headache clinics.

If you need or wish, this extension of biobehavioral therapy can take you deeply into your own perspective on the world, your pattern of relating, your history, or the operation of your current social structure. How far you go is, in the end, up to you. Your therapist will offer you his or her opinion about the need to address certain areas for long-term effectiveness of treatment. Even in your evaluation the psychologist may suggest areas that clearly need this type of attention. However, biobehavioral treatment is not an all-or-nothing affair. It is designed like a streetcar line; you can get off at any point, and you will have come some distance. What you have done to date will not be wasted effort even if you are not ready to go far on this particular extension of biobehavioral therapy or to get on it at all.

You will find that cognitive-behavioral therapy is ideally suited to a collaborative process between therapist and patient. You really can participate actively in care, so this chapter presents various techniques to help you assess and manage psychosocial stressors. In most cases you will be using these techniques as part of your overall biobehavioral management of headaches, so we assume that you will have a therapist to work on them with. In this way they will be useful in enriching the therapy process, and your therapist will help you make them specifically effective for you.

LEVEL ONE: RECOGNIZING AND CHANGING BEHAVIOR AND ATTITUDES

The first level of cognitive-behavioral therapy involves identifying your recurring psychosocial stressors and developing more effective, less tension-producing responses to them. This process began with the evaluations themselves, continued with the indirect effects of relaxation training and recordkeeping, and accelerated in your effort to generalize relaxation. At this point you have made some gains in managing headaches and are able to look at these recurring and resistant stressors more directly. As you do so, you will better determine their nature and what you might do differently when you encounter them. Here we will give the general categories of recurring stressors and just a few examples of each. Take the idea and work it out in more detail with your therapist.

Some stressors can simply be avoided. Like foods that trigger headaches, there are some people that you just don't have to include in your regular social "diet." There may be some guilt or social pressure, but you are not required to get along with everyone. Not every possible challenge in your life needs to be confronted either. There is no law that says you cannot avoid some battles when the greater good does not require them. If a particular line of work is not suited to your talents, perhaps now is not the time to prove that you can do it. However, as we know only too well, many (perhaps most) stressful situations cannot be eliminated so easily. Perhaps you find that your moral and social responsibility requires you to respond to a difficult family member, or you are not ready to take the consequences of leaving a secure job at this time. In that case you must consider what can change.

When you think of change, the first and most reliable place to look is in yourself. This may seem unfair, and you may wonder, *Why is it always I who must adapt?* Asking this question in itself may, however, suggest an area for exploration at the second stage of cognitive-behavioral therapy. For the moment, consider the idea that rather than being a burden the idea of looking to yourself for change is an invitation to greater independence. When you must rely on others to change for you to feel better, you lose (not gain) control. You have no real control over what others do. The belief that you can control others is one of the great illusions that brings much heartache.

Change in yourself may involve learning a new skill or way of thinking or improving an existing one. If you are often tense in social situations, consider the root of that tension. Do you have difficulty making conversation or worry a great deal about how others perceive you? If so, learning to make small talk or to ask others about themselves may move you toward greater social ease. If you can do so, it will reduce the tension and therefore the need to use relaxation in such situations.

Take another example. Do you feel overwhelmed at work, always seeming to get a new assignment even before you have finished the previous one? Despite all your efforts, does it seem that you are not recognized by the people who count? Then consider the possible underlying cause. Perhaps you'll find that you're not very assertive at work. If you can't discuss the situation with your boss, you will never know if he or she is just uncaring or simply has not noticed how hard you are working and how stressed you feel. Learning to be assertive is a valuable skill. It really boils down to learning how to be respectfully honest about yourself and informed about others. As you identify areas in which you need to add or improve a skill, your therapist will help you learn by reading, talking, rehearsing, and trying it out in "real life."

In other situations you will find the need to reduce or eliminate some ways of acting or thinking. For example, if you find yourself almost constantly angry, irritable, resentful, or sad, maybe your own view of the world needs to be changed. There are times in all our lives when such feelings are perfectly appropriate to the situation, but in most of our lives there is a balance. If you don't find one, you may be carrying your reality around with you, from the inside. You will be asked to take a look at the way you see situations and to consider alternative ways of seeing the same events or interpreting the intentions of others. Trying out new responses, even when at first they seem to be phony, may be the beginning of a new outlook, lightening the burden of a constantly negative mood and reducing a factor that contributes to headaches. The support of your therapist will be sustaining to you as you risk the new pattern of thinking and acting.

These are just a few examples of the kinds of situations you might encounter and the responses you might be called on to make. They are of necessity oversimplified, but they should illustrate the process by which you identify recurring sources of stress, analyze them to determine why they are getting to you, and develop a strategy for effectively resolving them.

Now we come to the flies in the ointment. The first is that on occasion, despite the many possibilities for modifying thoughts and behaviors that make stressors more troublesome, some stressors just cannot be avoided. The most obvious are the external and biological stressors, like weather and menstrual changes. However, this is also true of psychosocial stressors. In talks on this subject we use a slide that reads, "Please don't tell me to relax; my tension is the only thing holding me together." This little saying and the humorous cartoon of a figure held together with springs that accompanies it illustrate an important point. Life is difficult.

Sometimes we face events or periods in our life that are inherently stressful. At those times we can only rely on the realization that our stressful response is normal and on the relief that occurs when others willingly share the burden with us. This might be the role of family, friends, spiritual guide, or therapist. Laughter or light humor appropriate to the situation is one of the best tension-reducing responses. It arises most naturally from a spiritual or philosophical perspective on the stressful situation. Even appreciation, without denying the pain, may be possible. If you are able to look for the meaning in each situation or person you encounter, you are not likely to feel bounced around randomly by an uncaring fate.

An attitude of acceptance may seem foreign to many in our active culture, but it is often the most honest and active response we can make. There is little honor in continuing to bruise a bloodied head against an unyielding wall. At the very least, take the time to reassess the strategies you are using. The reward of honest and appropriate acceptance is the sense of calm and peace that accompanies it, quite compatible with the goal of generalizing relaxation. If the stressor is recurrent, it helps to remember that you can at least cushion yourself against the expected blow and prefer this option to trying to deny the reality and being caught unaware over and over again.

◆ THE CASE OF KAREN L., PART 6

During Karen L.'s initial evaluations her psychologist tentatively identified Karen as a very assertive, ambitious go-getter. So it was not surprising that she had difficulty finding time to practice relaxation when she began that mode of therapy. She also noticed that during relaxation practice she would often become impatient and that her mind would drift to problems at work. She worked with these problems with her therapist but then found, as she tried to generalize relaxation, that she seldom remembered to check for tension or try brief relaxation at work. Only near the end of the day, when her head was likely to be hurting, did she reflect on what had been happening. In conversations with her therapist Karen agreed that she demanded a lot of herself, but she had trouble deciding where to draw the line. It all seemed so natural. She liked her work and took pride in her ability to exceed most of the expectations held by her supervisors. In fact *not* pushing herself to achieve her goals seemed more stressful, and it was even worse when she asked someone less perfectionistic to help her! Karen agreed that she "wanted it all." She still saw the headaches as an imposition, cramping her style. Just talking about these traits and behaviors allowed Karen to reaffirm her recognition that the headaches were part of her, whether she liked it or not, and must be accommodated in some way if she was to enjoy her life. She could see that she had to make some changes.

The difficulty was in making these changes without losing her sense of competence and confidence. Some changes were easier to make than others. She approached her children, asking them to help more reliably with home responsibilities, which she had been trying to handle on her own. She also proposed to them that they set aside some time each week simply to enjoy each other in some mutually agreeable activity. Others were harder. She sat down with her boss, telling her that she felt overwhelmed by her current load although she recognized that she had taken on much of it herself. She could not have been more surprised when her boss replied that she had been concerned herself that Karen was going to "burn out." She turned out to be very helpful to Karen in reassessing her work, setting priorities, and delegating some tasks. Her family responded very well. They were not "perfect," of course, but they did feel more involved in her life, both by helping and by having some "quality time" with Karen.

These were big steps for Karen—setting limits on how much responsibility she would agree to take on and asking for help from others when she needed to. Karen's therapist facilitated the therapy process by taking a gentle and respectful approach. It was not the therapist's intention to take responsibility for Karen's choices. Rather the therapist wanted to help Karen recognize the choices she was making and to see their consequences more clearly. Once she did this, Karen could determine whether these choices were consistent with her most important values, were working for her overall good, and were leading to real control over her headaches.

LEVEL TWO: EXPLORING THE SOURCES OF BEHAVIOR AND ATTITUDES

For many headache sufferers the first stage of cognitive-behavioral therapy is sufficiently effective. They avoid the stressors that can be avoided, change their responses to those that cannot be avoided, and at least anticipate stressors when all else fails. But sometimes therapist and patient reach an impasse. (An impasse should be distinguished from situations in which treatment team and patient carry everything out according to plan but fail to see the expected decrease in headache frequency. Fortunately, this outcome is very rare, but when it occurs the first assumption is that something has been missed in the evaluation and treatment planning. The old phrase "back to the drawing board" applies well.)

Impasse refers to the situation in which the patient sees what must be done but does not carry it out. This may occur early in treatment, with the patient not practicing relaxation or becoming paradoxically anxious when trying to relax. More often, though, it occurs later in treatment, when working with recurring stressors. This is the second fly in the ointment. Some patients desire to make the behavioral changes suggested and work faithfully at this yet seem to make no steady progress. Perhaps the patient-therapist discussion made perfect sense in the office, but the patient was then unable to act on it during the week. In many cases matters go well for a time, but then the old way of thinking or acting returns in force. As soon as the pattern is recognized, the wise therapist does not continue simply to admonish or encourage the patient but suggests that they both back up to take a second and broader look at what is happening.

At the second stage of cognitive-behavioral therapy you and the therapist begin to dig deeper, below superficial appearances, for the obstacles to carrying out the biobehavioral therapy (or even the physical therapy or medication regimen) as suggested. Three basic questions are commonly considered to try to explain what, on the surface, appears to be self-defeating behavior. In the present situation, with the therapist or some other important person, is an issue from the past being acted out? In the present situation, is the person pursuing other goals that are incompatible with the goals established for taking control of headaches? Are the behavioral changes being attempted essentially incompatible with deeply ingrained patterns of behavior (or the individual's personality style)?

Let's look at a particular, and not unusual, example: a chronic headache sufferer feels overmatched and stuck in a relationship with a parent-in-law.

✦ THE CASE OF STEVEN S.

Steven S. suffered from frequent tension-type headaches. He had made progress in reducing their frequency from nearly every day to several per week. He and his therapist identified arguments with his father-in-law as a reliable and regular trigger of headaches. In analyzing the situation, they found that Steven's lack of assertiveness and apparent inability to leave the situation both severely exacerbated the stressfulness of the situation. In the therapist's office Steven worked to increase assertiveness skills, build self-esteem, and identify the very early stages of the usual arguments so that he might calm himself and change the direction of the conversation. In theory these changes should have helped Steven feel more effective in his relationship with the father-in-law, reduce the number of arguments, more quickly resolve arguments that do occur, and, as a result, reduce the tension that leads to a headache.

Unfortunately, when he and his father-in-law were together, Steven used none of these skills. Steven wanted to speak up to his father-in-law in an assertive manner, sticking to his own feelings and perceptions without attacking, but he just couldn't seem to do so. He just took his father-in-law's abusive language, started yelling, or did both in sequence. Even when he walked away from an argument, he stormed away, building his own anger, which seethed for hours afterward. His distress was increased by the headache that almost invariably followed this scene and his sense of embarrassment at not being able to do what he knew would be in his best interest.

Steven's therapist did not want to become just another player in this repeated drama. She could easily have become another abusing person by badgering Steven to use what he had learned. Instead she asked him to consider with her what was happening. She pointed out that he was continuing to act in the same way in spite of the skills he had developed and the plans he had made in his biobehavioral therapy. Her question was not accusing but evocative. What could be happening that led to this outcome that didn't seem to make sense?

In this case the answers were found in Steven's history of physical abuse at the hands of his own father. To cope with this very difficult situation, Steven had learned deeply ingrained habits of timid behavior in the face of aggressive men. Only when provoked beyond his tolerance would he lash out. At such times the violence of his verbal behavior frightened him as much as or more than the aggressiveness of the other. This pattern made it even more difficult for him to be assertive in the future. Even mild expressions of anger seemed risky to him. The anger did not go away, of course, but seethed within him. This suppressed anger contributed to depression and even lower self-esteem. For Steven to work through this situation, his therapist had to help him examine and talk about this history and how it was partly re-created in the arguments with his father-in-law. As he did so, he was better able to let the past be past and, even though the old issues were not yet worked out, understand the present situation more accurately for what it was. He found the courage to speak up and was pleased by the sense of respect he felt for himself, from others in the family, and even (grudgingly) from his father-in-law. None of this could have happened had his therapist not been aware of the possibility of deeper roots for apparently uncooperative and self-defeating behavior. If she had only pushed him to do more, he would have had at best another failure experience.

In this case the answer was found in an early life experience and in the very ingrained behavior pattern that Steven had developed. It could as easily have been in less obvious aspects of the situation itself. Very often, when there is apparently self-defeating behavior, there are competing goals that leave the person in conflict. For example, it may be that Steven would have had dependency needs that were as strong as his desire to reduce headache frequency. If the family expected everyone to cater to the father-in-law, standing up to his father-in-law would have meant risking rejection by the family. In that case the therapist might have suggested family therapy to get at the source of the impasse.

As we've noted, how far you go in this second phase of cognitive-behavioral therapy depends entirely on your situation and your desire. Most headache patients require only the first phase, approximately eight weekly sessions followed by less frequent sessions over the next few months in our experience. By the end you may be coming only about once per month, primarily to ensure that you have indeed gotten to the heart of the matter and are learning to maintain the changes you've made. For other patients longer therapy may be recommended. This may be offered through the headache clinic, or referral may be suggested to a psychologist or psychiatrist specializing in psychotherapy or family therapy. If that recommendation is made, you are still responsible for choosing whether you will act on it—then, later, or not at all. You still will have benefited from biobehavioral therapy, even if you do not continue as far as might be recommended.

A critical factor is your openness to psychological factors from the start. As we mentioned earlier in the book, some patients come with beliefs that the need for psychological assistance is a sign of personal weakness or somehow makes the headaches less "real." This attitude makes it just that much harder to plan and provide multimodal treatment. If you are reluctant to consider questions about your personal history and psychosocial situation or hold back information that may shed light on psychosocial triggers of your headache, you will undermine the team's ability to provide the biobehavioral portion of comprehensive therapy for your headache. We hope the information we have provided in these chapters will help you approach the psychological factors in your headache problem with courage, honesty, and a sound idea of the way they interact with physical factors to form your particular chronic headache syndrome.

✦ THE CASE OF KAREN L., CONCLUSION

Earlier in this chapter we explained that Karen did very well at learning relaxation skills in her therapist's office but had trouble remembering to use them in the course of her day, especially at work or school. Karen had learned the technique but was not generalizing it. Her therapist responded on several levels. The first addressed her problems with remembering and being willing to take the time for relaxation itself. The second addressed some of the habitual attitudes and behaviors that maintained the vicious circle of increased activity and heightened arousal. With attention, encouragement, and a willingness to take risks, Karen made several changes.

The first level of cognitive-behavioral therapy had allowed Karen to recognize many of the behaviors that increased her headache risk and to develop some options for change. However, Karen recognized that she was having real difficulty sticking with this arrangement. She felt uncomfortable when work was not done as she would have done it and still was drawn to the temporary "high" when she worked through a large and demanding project, even though the stress level was also high and time with her family was sacrificed. This strong need to achieve beyond all reason was a deeper issue, with roots in her own past. Getting at the source of this strong need was the focus of the next stage of cognitive-behavioral therapy.

This phase involved exploration of some of the deeper sources of Karen's great investment in achieving, even when it was interfering with family life, personal time, and headache management. She and her therapist discussed her reactions to limiting her work or allowing others to help. Even as they discussed her reactions, the therapist noticed that Karen seemed to slightly elevate her left shoulder; EMG increased at these times. The tensing was not something of which Karen was conscious, but it was very consistent. Karen and her therapist worked both to relax the muscles and to determine what thoughts and feelings were present at that time. They found two things that seemed very important.

First, Karen could recall that even from an early age she had been the "responsible" one in the family. She had taken care of other family members, sometimes even her parents. Even while she was still in grade school she seemed often to be more parent than child. Everyone appreciated this effort, and even neighbors and church members spoke of how "grown up" she was. She seemed to take the role naturally, rather than considering it a burden. Nevertheless, all this was taking its toll on her body.

Second, she began to see that this basic pattern had been exacerbated when she was divorced. Even in her marriage she had been the one who took the lead on most projects. After her divorce she felt even more pressure as a single mother and primary support of the family. Her way of coping was to throw herself into the challenge of her work and to take classes to advance herself.

This subject was not always easy for Karen to talk about. However, by this time she had a very trusting relationship with her biobehavioral therapist. She knew that the information would not be shared beyond the treatment team. In addition, as she spoke of these issues, it seemed to become easier for her to look at her situation freshly. She really began to believe that her competence was not in question and that she did not have to do more than her share to be sure of keeping her job. She began to take satisfaction not only from her work but also from the balance she could achieve in her life among work, school, family, and self. She found interests in herself that she never knew existed. In the process it was much easier to work with the generalization of basic relaxation as well, and headache frequency dropped further still.

Once again, we must emphasize the gentle approach of the therapist. Karen's therapist did not want to question the legitimacy of her feelings or urge her immediately to give up the satisfaction she got from work. To do so would only have exchanged one problem for another. Rather the therapist's job was to help Karen see more clearly the self-defeating pattern of her behavior and to help her understand what perspective was leading her to act in this way. From there Karen could consider more freely whether another way of looking at and handling the situation might be more effective. In fact she did find such a perspective that allowed her to maintain her sense of competence while taking better care of her body, mind, and spirit.

Karen was able to better appreciate her own value and lovableness, independent of how much she did for others. In this perspective her work seemed to spring from her own interests, energy, and vision rather than feeling like an imposition or requirement to be part of the "tribe." In addition, she began to see the coming together of others with their own talents and desires as a natural building up of the human family. Each member of a group—work, family, or others—supported the rest. She no longer felt "out on a limb" in carrying out her part.

Also once again, we must stress that it was the multimodal approach that helped Karen get to this point. It would be misleading to suggest that only more intensive relaxation training with biofeedback helped her extend relaxation into her daily life. It would even be misleading to say that the extensive cognitive-behavioral therapy was the key. Instead it was the combination of therapies—medical, physiological, and behavioral—that helped her resolve the headache syndrome. In her case is a small example of a comprehensive approach to headache treatment, one of the majority of cases in which multimodal therapy was effective in reducing the frequency and severity of a chronic, severe headache problem.

In presenting Karen's story over the span of several chapters in this book, each treating discrete aspects of multimodal treatment, we may have made the various aspects of comprehensive headache treatment seem more disjointed and separable than they really are. We have described separately the various aspects of care that actually occur simultaneously in an integrated treatment plan. We have categorized and phased in information and interventions that are applied much more flexibly, as they are needed, by the headache professionals on the treatment team. We have been able only to hint at the human touch that such doctors and therapists bring to their work. We hope, however, that presenting this information as we have has given you a clearer and more extensive understanding of how multimodal treatment works.

MAINTAINING THERAPEUTIC BENEFITS

Maintenance of the gains made during therapy is the final stage of treatment but not the least important. The responsibility for this stage falls largely on your shoulders, although for the first few months you may well have occasional visits with your biobehavioral therapist. You are likely to have periodic visits with your physician for a longer time. Maintaining the benefits of your therapy requires at least three things.

1. Practice What You Learned in Your Physical and Biobehavioral Therapy

Fortunately for most of us, this does not mean keeping up the level of practice that was required early in treatment. Over the course of therapy you should have made habitual the changes in posture and movement that were trained by physical therapy exercises. In biobehavioral therapy you have probably increased your reliance on brief relaxation and recognition of early signs of tension. This becomes the dominant mode of behavioral headache management after the active phase of care. Again, the frequency with which you practice the extended relaxation exercise will no doubt be reduced. Now an attitude of self-regulation should be incorporated into your way of planning your day, anticipating triggers of headache, recognizing conditions that create fertile ground for the development of headaches, and continuing to increase life satisfaction in the context of a healthy, balanced life. You can use the checklists in Appendix I, modified as necessary, to monitor your self-management during the follow-up period. This process of continuing to put it all together, gradually but consistently over time, is the ideal form of maintenance. It is the most appropriate complement for the comprehensive headache treatment in which you have participated.

2. *Continue to Accept That Your Headaches Are Chronic*

Remember that there is no current cure for chronic headaches. Because of this, no matter how successful your treatment has been, headaches will recur. Under the wrong conditions they may even become frequent again. Naturally, if you have an unusually severe headache, new symptoms, or suddenly frequent headaches, ask your physician first to review the diagnosis and assure you that no new disease is present. If there is no new medical diagnosis, review your current management against what you have learned. If you find that psychosocial or other triggers of headaches have increased in your life, make the move to reduce them. Do not fall prey to the incorrect assumption that the multimodal treatment did not work after all and avoid seeking more radical or unusual therapy as your response to a relapse.

3. *Feel Free to Call on Your Doctor and Therapist Again*

Many things can initiate a relapse. Big changes in your life or physical condition—relocating, changing jobs, receiving new medication, undergoing menopause, suffering an injury—may trigger a major flare-up of headaches. But even small changes can set up a gradually escalating circle of tension and increasing headache. They can be hard to spot.

If you cannot determine what has happened to increase headache frequency, ask your treatment team to see you again to evaluate current medication use, muscle state, relaxation practice, and behavioral stressors. If you have moved, ask them to recommend a headache clinic in your new area; your team will be glad to do so and to send along records of your previous treatment. With the history of your headaches and prior treatment in their files, your doctors and therapists will be more quickly able to suggest measures that will help you reestablish control of your headaches. And you, having maintained the benefits of your therapy by reviewing and practicing what you've learned, will be able to act constructively and respond decisively to their suggestions. You will again take control.

CHAPTER 10

✦

Special Categories of Headaches

In the preceding chapters we have tried to cover all the bases for most people who suffer from chronic or severe headaches. There are, however, a few categories of headaches that require special consideration in evaluation and treatment. If you have headaches associated with temporomandibular dysfunction (TMD) or your headaches arose following a head or neck injury, the multimodal evaluation and therapy we have described may be supplemented with additional evaluations or treatments and/or consultations by other specialists. However, recent research has shown that these classes of headaches lend themselves well to multidisciplinary treatment.

Throughout this book we have stressed that chronic headaches can plague just about anyone. That includes people from six to sixty (and beyond), and while the methods covered here apply to headache sufferers of all ages, the very young and the elderly sometimes have special requirements. Part of this chapter is devoted to telling you how those needs can be met by the multimodal approach to treatment and how you can get the help you deserve from your health care team.

HEADACHES FOLLOWING HEAD OR NECK TRAUMA

According to the National Head Injury Foundation, a head injury (trauma) occurs in the United States about every fifteen seconds. Many of these occur as a result of motor vehicle accidents. Headaches are a common symptom of such head injuries. Frequently these injuries are minor, and the headaches disappear within a few months at most. But in some cases the symptoms, including headaches, persist for much longer, perhaps for years. Long-lasting headache following mild head injury may occur in as many as 30 percent of all cases. In most of these cases standard medical examination reveals no treatable physical cause for the headaches. Still, the pain persists.

We know that chronic headaches following head or neck trauma are not restricted to one type; they may take the form of any of the major chronic headache types. The patient often shows evidence of muscle irritation—stiffness, tenderness, restriction of movement—in the neck, upper back, and/or facial areas. The headaches may increase in frequency over time. The patient also often suffers from depression, suppressed anger, and/or anxiety. This psychological distress is a reflection of several factors, including the effects of the accident itself, the prolonged pain, and unsuccessful efforts to get treatment. Unfortunately, these feelings then further exacerbate the headache syndrome.

If you are in this situation, it is likely that your primary physician and consulting physicians have invested considerable effort into trying to determine the cause of your headaches. Both you and your physicians have probably been frustrated by the failure of this effort to uncover definite causes or by the failure of medication and other treatments, usually applied one at a time, to end the headaches. Perhaps you have now resorted to using more medication than you think is good for you and are still finding little benefit from it. You may feel that your physician is responding skeptically to your report of continuing headache pain. You may wonder if the doctor thinks you are merely seeking drugs or trying to postpone returning to work. You may even have gotten into the unfortunate position of becoming defensive about your psychological distress for fear that your headaches will be interpreted as a psychological problem only. At this point you are in the same position that we have described for chronic headache patients in general.

The good news is that chronic headache following head injury can often be treated just as successfully as the frequent severe headaches without any such trauma. It is not unusual to find that the multimodal approach to evaluation will allow physician, physical therapist, and psychologist to set up a comprehensive treatment plan with a good chance of success. Just receiving a clear explanation for your headaches helps a great deal. As you have seen elsewhere in this book, muscle irritation can be a powerful trigger of headaches, and muscle irritation is a common result of head and neck trauma. The psychological distress resulting from the accident or from the pain itself must also be addressed directly to reduce its role in prolonging headache. Subtle changes in the ability to think clearly or to recall information can be diagnosed with testing, and strategies can be developed to compensate for them. Finally, over a period of prolonged headache it is not unusual for medication use to increase to the point of causing rebound headache, yet another treatable factor in prolonged headaches after trauma. Of course, the possibility of an undiscovered medical cause for the headaches is always considered in the medical portion of multimodal treatment and continues to be considered if you do not respond to treatment as expected.

HEADACHES ASSOCIATED WITH TEMPOROMANDIBULAR DYSFUNCTION

Perhaps you have read about or consulted a physician or dentist about facial pain associated with temporomandibular dysfunction. If so, you know that such problems are often associated with pain around the ears, at the joint by which the jaw moves, in front of the face where you usually think of sinus pain, in the lower jaw, in the teeth, or in the temple. This type of pain is often aggravated by chewing, clenching, or grinding the teeth. It is a recurring disorder, worsening and then improving over time for no discernible reason in many people.

What you may not know is that this is probably not a single disorder. There are many explanations from different practitioners (and many names for the disorder!), but it has been hard to get a single explanation that satisfies every case. In a very few individuals the reason for the problem is in the very poor arrangement of the teeth, requiring orthodontic care like braces. In some it seems that the problem is due to a disturbance of the joint (temporomandibular joint) itself. In many more patients part of the problem, or even its primary source, is irritation of the muscles that move the jaw. This irritation, as discussed earlier in the book, may be associated with habitual postures or movements that overuse the muscles, in this case the jaw muscles.

One of the common symptoms associated with temporomandibular dysfunction—also called *myofascial pain, craniomandibular disorder,* or *TMJ*—is chronic headache. When the pain remains in one of the areas noted above, often on one side of the head, we call it *local pain.* However,

TMD often seems to act as a trigger of recognizable chronic headache syndromes. In our experience the local pain and irritation of TMD can be identified as a trigger of tension-type or migraine headache. This is a very common finding among people who have chronic headache following head or neck trauma.

This does not mean that the headache is "really" TMD. The important thing to remember is that in chronic severe headache we try to take a comprehensive look at the problem. If TMD is present, it may be part of the problem, and therefore it must be treated. However, when a recognizable headache syndrome is present, TMD and its treatment should still be considered *part* of the overall evaluation and treatment plan. When the treatments are coordinated, there is less likelihood that money and time will be wasted and a greater chance that the treatments used can be applied to both problems simultaneously.

In particular, it is important not to accept as the first line of treatment the irreversible treatments that might be suggested by some practitioners. These might include grinding the teeth, pulling teeth, or performing surgery on the temporomandibular joint. In most cases first-stage treatment of even severe TMD (with or without headaches as a symptom) will involve the integrated application of physical therapy (often a part of the headache treatment plan in any case), biobehavioral therapy (to eliminate habits of muscle overuse and address psychosocial stressors), and an oral appliance fashioned by a dentist experienced in this area. The appliance itself is often a simple device to change the relationship of the upper and lower jaw, reducing habitual tension of the muscles. It may also take pressure off the temporomandibular joint when it is painfully irritated. More radical treatment should usually be reserved for cases in which these therapies do not help.

HEADACHES AT A LATER AGE

Elderly is a subjective term. The age by which you become elderly varies according to several factors, including how old you happen to be today and how you are feeling! When we speak of headaches, *older* certainly means sixty-five years and beyond. Some writers will begin to think of people as older at fifty-five or even after menopause.

There are at least two reasons for a special section on headaches among older people. First, the common wisdom among many health professionals is that headaches are not a significant problem after menopause or for the elderly. Headaches and their treatment in older individuals have been topics of much less study than for younger people. While it is true that migraine headaches decrease steadily among older people taken as a group, they still occur in some. If you have migraine headaches, you deserve to have it diagnosed and treated appropriately, no matter what your age. In addition, other forms of headache, particularly tension-type headaches, continue to be a relatively common symptom among older people. While they rarely develop after age sixty, they often persist from an earlier period of your life. Cluster headaches too strike older adults.

Second, as our bodies age, we handle medications differently. Some prescriptions for common headache medications are no longer permissible because of other disease. Other medicines must be given in lower doses to avoid side effects. Also, once you reach your later years you are more likely to be taking a variety of drugs for a variety of conditions (and sometimes from a variety of doctors), which can easily interact with medications that might be prescribed for headaches.

As with any headache, diagnosis is the first and the ongoing concern. If you are experiencing new or worsened headaches, seek evaluation first from your primary care physician. He or she usually can coordinate the most comprehensive assessment. Consultation from a physician specializing in geriatric and/or headache medicine may be requested by your physician. Among older adults, headaches are more often a sign of serious and complex disease than they are among younger people. They may also be the result of medications you are taking for other reasons. Hormonal changes are a common factor in headaches among younger individuals. While the onset of menopause often signals a reduction in headache frequency, it does not do so universally. Some headaches begin or become worse after menopause, and hormone replacement therapy must always be considered among the possible factors for headaches in older persons.

Among the more benign factors that may trigger or contribute to headaches, you must consider all the trigger and contributing factors discussed earlier in this book. Any of them could be playing a role now. In this section we can give only a few examples.

Posture and repetitive movements may lead to stiff and sore muscles. These should not be considered an inevitable consequence of aging and can still be addressed productively in physical therapy and biobehavioral therapy. We often slow down with age, but that should not be seen as a reason to stop exercise altogether. If you have become much less active, consider engaging in a progressive exercise program, especially for older people, after medical clearance. Regular exercise will help reduce the headache problem just as in younger people. You will also feel better generally.

How well do you sleep? As we age, sleep can be interrupted by a variety of factors, including sleep disorders, medication side effects, and depression. Poor quality of sleep and insufficient amount of sleep are risk factors now as they were earlier in life.

We speak euphemistically of old age as the "golden years," but some people tell us they seem more rusty than golden. Regardless of how much we might look forward to retirement, grandchildren, and pursuing those avocations we never had time for, aging brings psychosocial stressors that can contribute to headache risk. Even fit bodies decline in function; illnesses occur more often. Injury or disease may lead to physical impairment. There are fundamental changes in relationships as spouse, family members, or friends die. Any of these losses may prove difficult to manage, and poorly managed losses may lead to depression, not uncommon among the elderly.

Aging is not automatically associated with depression and disability. Many older people live actively, pursuing their interests for many years. However, if life is difficult, the older years are an advanced challenge. Success does not come without awareness, planning, and activity. This applies as well to taking control of your headaches. You must deal even more effectively with the physical, mental, and spiritual challenges of aging to reduce headache risk. But remember that your headache problem is as worthy of attention now as when you were younger. You can get effective help in assessing and responding to the problem with more than just more pills.

Examine yourself also to see if you have any dysfunctional attitudes that are making you your own worst enemy. Do you believe you should just be able to put up with the pain? Do you worry that you are making too much of your headaches? Such stoicism is not unusual among the elderly. Are you embarrassed to press your doctor for an effective response when no medical disease is found to explain the headache? Do you worry that psychological factors affecting your headache make you "crazy"? Clinging to such beliefs only leaves you with pain that can prevent you from living the active, satisfying life you deserve.

It's in your interest, then, to tell your doctor about all your concerns, to answer questions honestly, and to remember that you can be treated effectively for your headache pain. There is no shame in expressing worries you may have about your diagnosis or in asking for more thorough and multimodal evaluation. Be open with your doctor about the effect of your pain on your life. Try to be open to family or friends who may suggest that you are taking too much medicine or may wonder if you would do well to talk with a psychologist. Say so if you want more time from your doctor or a clearer explanation of evaluation and treatment recommendations. If he or she does not respond appropriately to such requests, it is not your problem; seek another doctor.

HEADACHES AMONG CHILDREN

Another group in which many people do not expect to find headaches is children. For reasons not entirely clear, severe headaches often have not been diagnosed and treated adequately in children, particularly in preteens. Too often children complaining of headaches have been dismissed as trying to avoid school or other responsibilities. In fact, however, frequent severe headaches are found among children. Migraine headaches may be harder to recognize because among younger children they often do not include all of the common diagnostic indicators found in adults. Most of the triggers that can affect headaches in adults are also possible in children, including muscle irritation, dietary triggers, and psychosocial stress.

As we noted earlier, susceptibility to chronic headaches seems to run in families; if you are reading this book because you have severe headaches, be alert for them in your child. Although it is not impossible, it is not likely that you will promote such complaints from your child by your attention to them. In any case, complaints of severe pain that are truly motivated by ulterior motives will be evident only over time. For children with chronic headache there is no reason to withhold quality multidisciplinary evaluation and treatment similar to that offered to adults.

Naturally, complaints of severe headaches should lead first to diagnosis. Consult your child's pediatrician. He or she may also ask the opinion of a pediatric neurologist or other consultant. If your child has complained of frequent severe headaches, and such diagnosis has not produced any significant medical findings, ask about the availability of a comprehensive headache clinic that will accept children for multimodal evaluation and treatment.

The good news is that the type of treatment described in this book for adults can be quite effective, with appropriate modifications, for even young children. In fact children may actually be more adept at learning and using the biobehavioral therapy we've described. Children are adept at learning relaxation, visualization, and deep breathing, and they quickly learn to identify triggers and modify physical, cognitive, and behavioral responses to them. In many cases their treatment is briefer than that of adults.

Children are capable of taking a great deal of responsibility for their own headache management. The general course of treatment is exactly as we have described; however, evaluation and treatment must be adapted to the age of the child. If your child is too young to have developed the verbal ability to describe symptoms and emotions fully, the treatment team may use modified recording forms, emphasizing simple scales, drawings, and expressive faces children can point to. Adult relaxation exercises and audiotapes for home practice may not be as helpful with young children. Special or even individualized tapes are often provided. Young children will also need parental assistance in learning and applying the relaxation.

Treatment for children necessarily includes the parents. The child's environment is so dominated by the home, and secondarily by the school, that it is not productive to attempt treatment without assessment of these settings and the involvement of important persons. What's happening in the family and at school with teachers and peers may be understood by the treatment team as psychosocial stress factors leading to internal tension and heightened risk of headache. Parents may have critical roles in placing limits on activity, avoiding unintentional reinforcement of "sick role" behavior, and reducing contributing factors like poor diet, poor sleep habits, overuse of medication, or physical inactivity. Whatever the age of the child, the team will depend a great deal on your observations as parents. Discrepancies between the child's report of pain and the observed behavior may lead to a clearer understanding of psychological factors. For example, a child or teenager who reports severe pain but is observed to be listening to loud music may be understood differently from one who is restricted to bed and asks for quiet.

Parents often sit in for part of the treatment session. The child explains what he or she has learned that day and describes the assignments for the week. The therapist buttresses the description of home exercises in relaxation or muscle stretching and strengthening. The parents report their own observations and ask whatever questions have arisen. When indicated, family therapy may be part of the treatment process. If needed, it is important that you not avoid this recommendation because you don't want to be exposed or involved. It is important for the child's recovery, but it is probably just as important for you and your family. Sometimes headaches can be a symptom of family disturbance as much as of the individual's physical and psychological state.

♦

Postscript

In this book, we have tried to bring you both hope and knowledge. We wanted to inspire you with the hope that your chronic headache problem can be treated. We know from prior studies that far too many people who have frequent severe headaches suffer alone. Most have tried to seek treatment at least once, some several times, but without success. They may continue to look for answers, emerging periodically from their solitary suffering with the dimmest of hopes, or they may just try to manage on their own.

If you are one of this number, you know well enough your own reasons for discouragement. Perhaps you felt that no one understood your problem. Maybe it seemed that your physician did not believe you had serious pain or did not seem to have time for you. Perhaps you got the impression that he or she thought you were only seeking drugs. You may have heard explanations that attributed the whole headache problem to psychological stress or to your inability to tolerate pain. Ultimately you might have come to believe that your physician did not have the answers to your problem, so you directed yourself in a series of sporadic visits to various medical specialists or other professionals. In this irregular and self-guided effort to find help you may have tried many or all of the therapies discussed in this book—and more—one at a time, without benefit.

We hope that reading this book has encouraged you to try again. Informed as you now are, and in collaboration with your primary care physician and the specialists of a comprehensive headache clinic, you have an extremely good chance of taking control of your headaches through an organized multimodal approach to treatment. You can expect not only to reduce the frequency of your headaches but also to limit the severity of the headaches you do have.

What kind of knowledge have we given you? Certainly we have not pretended to offer exhaustive treatment of all the different types of headaches and how they produce pain. Nor was there space in this book to cover each possible mode of treatment in great depth. And, we'll say it again, this book is not meant to substitute for the individualized professional treatment you deserve and can get at a comprehensive headache clinic.

Our desire in this book has been to bring you knowledge of how to find the help you need, of what makes effective treatment for frequent severe headache, of how to do your part in this treatment, of how to *make it work* rather than seeing if it will.

Taking control of chronic headaches is usually not a matter of finding the one reason you have headaches or the single magic treatment that will end them. Real and effective treatment of frequent severe headaches is more than taking a pill—or many pills. Until the day scientific medicine makes sufficient advances to find cause and cure for such headaches, frequent severe headaches are best considered a chronic medical illness and treated with a combination of effective therapies. These therapies can be selected rationally on the basis of existing research, clinical experience, and comprehensive evaluation of the special factors affecting your particular headache.

It is this rational process of evaluation and therapy that we have tried to share in this book. Evaluation and therapy can and should be individualized to fit you; there is no reason to think that a "one size fits all" program will give you the help you need. Your treatment plan should be flexible, changing in response to your observations and your response. An individualized and flexible plan of treatment, designed by a team of experts and implemented collaboratively with you, is the best way to ensure that your condition improves and that you maintain those improvements.

Finally, remember that your need for knowledge does not end here. You will continue to learn from your primary care physician, the comprehensive headache treatment team, your own observations, and the other books we recommend at the back of this book. Before, during, and after your period of active treatment, we also suggest you take advantage of the educational services offered by the National Headache Foundation and ACHE, whose phone numbers are listed in Chapter 1.

We sincerely desire your return to a fuller life, based on the recognition that you must take responsibility for managing your headaches, but nurtured in the realization that you can do so without letting headaches become the main focus of your living. With your open mind and active reading, we hope this book has brought you the hope and knowledge that will send you on your way to the help that is available to you. Godspeed and good fortune in taking control of your headaches.

✦

Checklists for Self-Help

A s Chapter 5 explained, your doctors at a comprehensive headache clinic are likely to ask you to keep a diary when you first consult them. This diary allows you to record information on your headaches, what triggers them, what contributing factors come into play for you, and more. Of necessity, it is usually a lengthy, detailed form. If you're not currently keeping such a diary, you can use the checklist in Chapter 5 for recording headache factors. You can also use the checklists given in this appendix. Checklist 1 is a simplified set of questions for keeping a daily diary; use it to keep track of your headaches. Checklist 2 is intended to encourage compliance with the treatment plan devised by your professional team and participation in self-care. Make several photocopies of each checklist so that you can use one copy each day.

You may find that these checklists include more detail than you need. At some point you may want to simplify, perhaps with the advice of your doctor or therapist, and come up with checklists specifically tailored to your unique situation.

CHECKLIST 1: A RECORD OF HEADACHES

Use this checklist to record information about your headaches themselves. This is important not only for diagnosis at the beginning of treatment—for which you may, as explained in Chapter 5, be asked to keep a more complete diary—but also to track changes in your headaches as treatment progresses. Make an entry for each headache (if intermittent) or each day (if headache seems continuous).

Date: _____

At what time did the headache occur? _____

How long did the headache last? _____

What was the maximum intensity of the headache on a scale of 1 (slight) to 10 (severe)? Draw a graph of headache intensity over the time pain lasted.

_____

_____

In what areas of head, face, and/or neck did headache pain occur?

_____

_____

What did the pain feel like (dull, throbbing, pounding, shooting, squeezing, boring, burning, etc.)?_____

_____

_____

Were there any other symptoms (nausea, visual effects, etc.)? _____

_____

_____

What factors might have been important in triggering this headache (see Chapter 5)? _____

_____

What did you do in trying to manage this headache? _____

_____

Note. Permission to reproduce this form is granted to purchasers of *Taking Control of Your Headaches* for personal use only.

CHECKLIST 2: FOLLOWING THROUGH ON TREATMENT

Date: _____

Below are statements you should recognize from Chapters 6–9 on the individual modes of headache treatment. Use a form like this to help you see how you are following through with the advice of your doctors and therapists or self-help techniques you have resolved to use on a regular basis.

Take prescribed medications in the proper dose at the proper time. (See Chapter 6.)			
Medication (list below)	Times of day taken	Dosage	Side effect

Use over-the-counter medications only as advised by your doctor. (See Chapter 6.)		
Medication (list below)	Times of day taken	Dosage

Practice physical therapy exercises. (See Chapter 7.)

Exercise (list below)   Times practiced   Repetitions

Extended relaxation:

Times practiced   Length of session   Effects

Brief relaxation:

Times practiced   Places practiced   Effects

Recognize and change behaviors that may
increase stress or interfere with treatment. (See Chapter 9.)

Behavior recognized (list) (describe)   Opportunity for change

---

✦

Controlling Headache Risk during Menstrual Periods

Despite the wide variation in how headaches and menstrual periods are related among women (described in Chapter 4), there are some steps that women can take before and during periods that should help control their risk of headache.

DIET

1. Eat smaller and more frequent meals.
2. Reduce fat intake.
3. Reduce caffeine (coffee, tea, cola, chocolate).
4. Reduce salt. See lists that follow.
5. Increase complex carbohydrates, such as crackers, bread, peas, rice, squash, pasta, beans, corn, potatoes.
6. Increase potassium, from foods such as milk, potatoes, asparagus, celery, apricots, grapes, bananas, carrots, broccoli, brussels sprouts, cauliflower.
7. Increase magnesium, from foods such as dark green vegetables, legumes, cereal grains, milk.
8. Ask your doctor about a mild diuretic, but be sure to maintain adequate water intake.
9. Limit alcohol intake.
10. Limit sweets—don't feed cravings.
11. Ask your doctor about vitamin supplements. This is a controversial area, so individually tailored advice from your doctor is advisable. In any case, you should ensure adequate intake of vitamins and minerals

in natural forms, including especially vitamins B6 and C, folate, iron, calcium, potassium, and magnesium.

EXERCISE

Exercise improves circulation and distribution of oxygen in your body. It helps eliminate body fluids and increases the production of endorphins, the body's natural painkillers. Below are described some exercises we feel may be especially helpful to women before and during menstrual periods.

To get the greatest benefit, go slowly—overly vigorous exercise may aggravate headaches. Be careful not to irritate neck, shoulder, or upper-back muscles. Review the suggestions that follow with your doctor or therapist to find the ones most appropriate for you.

1. Heads up. Strengthens abdominals, relieves back pressure. On back, knees bent, hands behind head: raise head, shoulders, and shoulder blades off the floor in that order, exhaling. Inhale as you lower shoulder blades first, then shoulders, and finally head.
2. Arm swing. Relieves midback tension. Standing, arms out from shoulders, make slow circles backward and then forward, both arms at the same time.
3. Pelvic rocking. Increases flexibility, strengthens abdominals, improves circulation. On back, knees bent, push low back to floor, then relax.
4. Knee and head roll. On back, knees bent, arms straight out from shoulders, roll knees to one side and head to opposite side.
5. Back stretch. Strengthens back and abdomen. On hands and knees, lower head and arch back. Exhale as you lower and arch. Then inhale as you lift head and return to original position.
6. Shoulder lifts and circles. Make circles forward and backward with shoulders, keeping arms at sides.

Walking, gentle aerobics, and swimming are all helpful for increasing strength, flexibility, and endurance. Don't push too hard, breathe slowly and easily, and never hold your breath while straining. Exercise should be relaxing!

OTHER AIDS DURING MENSTRUATION

1. Don't skimp on sleep. Keep regular hours.
2. Stop smoking.
3. Receive massage, especially to the upper back, neck, and shoulders.
4. Reduce stress at home and work.

5. Discuss your menstrual problems with family or others close to you.
6. Do relaxation exercises regularly.
7. Build up your coping skills. Think of symptoms as something to be worked with. Develop a sense of personal control appropriate to the situation. You don't have perfect control—there is no cure!—but you can influence things for the better.
8. Ask your doctor about a nonsteroidal anti-inflammatory medication for use prior to menstrual period to prevent headaches.

◆

Further Reading

BOOKS

Diamond, Seymour, Diane Frances, and Amy Diamond Vye. *Headache and Diet.* Madison, CT: International Universities Press, 1990.

Diamond, Seymour, and Mary Franklin, *Coping with Your Headaches.* Madison, CT: International Universities Press, 1982.

Hanh, Thich Nhat. *The Miracle of Mindfulness.* Boston: Beacon Press, 1987.

Kabat-Zinn, Jon. *Full Catastrophe Living.* New York: Dell, 1990.

Rapoport, Alan M., and Fred D. Sheftell. *Headache Relief.* New York: Simon & Schuster, 1990.

Saper, Joel, and Kenneth Magee. *Freedom from Headaches.* New York: Simon & Schuster, 1981.

Smith, Jonathan C. *Relaxation Dynamics.* Champaign, IL: Research Press, 1989.

Solomon, Seymour, and Steven Fraccaro. *The Headache Book: Effective Treatments to Prevent Headaches and Relieve Pain.* Mt. Vernon, NY: Consumer Reports Books, 1991.

Taddey, John, with Constance Schrader and James Dillon. *TMJ.* Surrey Park Press, 1990. Available from New Beginnings, P.O. Box 2887, La Jolla, CA 92038-2887.

AUDIOTAPES

Budzynski, Thomas. *Relaxation Training Program.* New York: Guilford Press, 1989.

Duckro, Paul N. *Gatherers at the Spring of Being* (with spiritual focus). Available from St. Louis Behavioral Medicine Institute, 1129 Macklind, St. Louis, MO 63110.

Duckro, Paul N. *Progressive Relaxation*. Available from St. Louis Behavioral Medicine Institute, 1129 Macklind, St. Louis, MO 63110.

VIDEOTAPES

No More Headaches. Xenejenex (in cooperation with National Headache Foundation). Catalog # XEN-74 (800-228-2495).

Relief from Migraine. Xenejenex (in cooperation with American Association for the Study of Headache). Catalog # XEN-76 (800-228-2495).

Index

◆

Letter to Professionals

Dear Health Care Professional:

Severe, frequent, and refractory headache can be frustrating not only for patients but the professionals who treat them as well. While medication is effective in most cases, its efficacy steadily decreases for some patients, who then run the risk of overusing both prescribed and over-the-counter medication. These patients are likely to benefit from the multidisciplinary treatment described in this book.

The program of care described here is found, in some form, in most major headache clinics. This approach cannot promise to cure headaches, but it can be effective in reducing their frequency and severity. Nevertheless, many patients with refractory headache syndromes are reluctant to be referred to clinics, and have trouble believing that treatments other than medication can really help.

This book stresses that headache remains a *real* medical disorder. In language the patient can understand and apply, we place medication in the broad context of potentially effective treatments and explain in detail the nature of multidisciplinary care for headache. Providing a hands-on introduction to biopsychosocial evaluation and treatment, we also consider the wide range of medical, neuromuscular, psychological, social, and dietary factors that can affect headache activity. We give special attention to the role of psychological and social factors that influence headache frequency and impact—concepts that are often the most difficult for patients to appreciate. By helping them understand, this book can remove a significant barrier to referral for multidisciplinary care.

Most difficult chronic headache syndromes can be effectively treated with multidisciplinary care. You play an important role in easing the process of referral for patients and opening the doors to effective treatment. We hope this book will make that task easier for you.

It can be used with patients in may ways. We suggest the following and hope that you will let us know of others.

- ✦ Primary care physicians can use it to introduce patients to the concept of multidisciplinary treatment prior to referral to a headache clinic or specialist.

- ✦ Headache specialists and their professional staffs can assign it as patient reading to reinforce the information they provide in treatment. The book can help to elicit important patient information and is designed to educate patients about the coordination necessary among professionals involved in a multidisciplinary treatment plan. It also serves as a patient reference and self-help guide when used within the treatment setting. Other books and tapes that are useful for this purpose are noted in the "Further Reading" section.

- ✦ Mental health care providers can use the book to correct patient misconceptions about the role of psychosocial factors in headache syndromes, thus paving the way for their active participation in multidisciplinary treatment.

If this book belongs to a colleague or patient, and you are interested in examining it in greater detail, the publisher is making a limited number of examination copies available to health care providers. You may call The Guilford Press toll-free at (800)365-7006 to receive your copy, which may be examined for 30 days with no obligation to purchase. Please also see the following two pages. They describe two methods for making this volume easily available to your patients.

Paul N. Duckro
William D. Richardson
Janet E. Marshall

Quantity Discounts and a Special Service for Recommending
Taking Control of Your Headaches

To the Health Care Professional:

Here are two convenient methods for ordering *Taking Control of Your Headaches.*

❶ QUANTITY DISCOUNTS

For multiple copies of *Taking Control of Your Headaches,* calculate the following discount rates against the list price to get the unit discount price. Then simply multiply the discount price times the quantity you are ordering. Add 5% of your total order for shipping.

QUANTITY	LIST PRICE	DISCOUNT	PRICE PER BOOK
1 book	$14.95	—	$14.95
2–12 books		20% off list price	$11.95
13–24 books		30% off list price	$10.45
25+		33% off list price	$9.85

To order, please call toll-free 1-800-365-7006

❷ PRIORITY ORDER FORMS

Or, when recommending the book, you may have individuals order directly from Guilford—simply photocopy the Priority Order Form on the next page. Priority Order Forms are given immediate attention.

We also assure confidentiality. Customers who use these order forms will be excluded from the Guilford mailing list and will receive no further correspondence.

We suggest that you also photocopy the order form for future use.

PRIORITY ORDER FORM

Send to: **Guilford Publications, Inc., Dept. IV**
72 Spring Street, New York, NY 10012

 CALL TOLL-FREE 1-800-365-7006
Mon.–Fri. , 9am–5pm EST
Or **FAX 212-966-6708**

(Be sure to tell the representative you are ordering from our Priority Order Form.)

NAME

ADDRESS

CITY   STATE   ZIP

DAYTIME PHONE NO.

Method of Payment

☐ Check or money order enclosed.

Please bill my   ☐ VISA   ☐ MasterCard   ☐ AmEx

ACCT. #

☐☐☐☐ ☐☐☐☐ ☐☐☐☐ ☐☐☐☐

Expiration Date: MONTH ☐☐ YEAR ☐☐

SIGNATURE

(required for all credit card orders)

Name of recommending professional:

Please Ship:

Qty.		Cat. #	Amount
1	Taking Control of Your Headaches	2787	$14.95
*Shipping Priority Mail—1 to 2 week delivery		Shipping*	$3.50
		NY and PA add sales tax	
		TOTAL	

PRIORITY ORDER
For office use only
Note: Operator—
set up as account type IT—
Mail <u>No</u>—Rush Order
SHIP VIA FC